WONDERS
OF A SINGLE DOSE
IN
HOMOEOPATHY

WONDERS
of a single dose
IN
HOMOEOPATHY

By
Dr. K. D. Kanodia

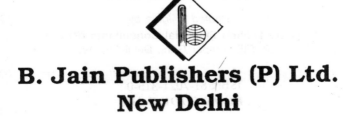

B. Jain Publishers (P) Ltd.
New Delhi

Price. Rs. 49.00

Reprint Edition: 2002, 2005

Published by

KULDEEP JAIN

for

B. Jain Publishers (P) Ltd.
1921, Chuna Mandi, St. 10th, Paharganj,
New Delhi-110 055
Ph: 2358 0800. 2358 1100. 2358 1300. 2358 3100
Fax: 011-2358 0471; *Email:* bjain@vsnl.com
Website: **www.bjainbooks.com**

Printed in India by
Unisons Techno Financial Consultants (P) Ltd.
522, FIE, Patpar Ganj, Delhi-110 092

ISBN 81-7021-315-0
BOOK CODE B-3368

PUBLISHER NOTE

Millians of pearls of wisdom are scattered over in the oceas of knowledge imparted by the pioneers of Homoeopathy. Nothing is original except the provings of drugs and their symptoms brought to light from time to time as also the clinical experiences highlighted by the master minds.

The requirement of the age is to assemble the technicalities in way that the pearls become useful as garlands and the people of wider sphere—
(a) the busy physicians (b) the learners, and (c) the educated masses - can study, understand and realise the blessings showered upon the human race by originator of this science.

The author's present work is a milistone in this direction and we feel confident that this will render the science more interesting, to study more practical to practice and more certain and fast for the results expected.

PUBLISHERS

CONTENTS

CONTENTS

PREFACE

Since 1810, when the natural law of healing was brought to light by Dr. Samuel Christian Fredrick Hahnemann, the science of homoeopathy (similia similibus curentur-Likes are cured by Likes) has much advanced.

Basically, homoeopathy restores the body to health by stimulating the healing forces within the body.

This volume of the compilation is to high light the achievements by renowned physicians of the world; to create a feeling of confidence and surely of results in this system; to acquaint the people and profession about the wonders of the drug in potency; and to impress upon all that it is the quickest and the safest system of restoring health.

Homoeopathy studies the plant life, animal life and the metals with all the aspects and background and establishes a relation to individual human life in particular condition. This co-relation and co-incidence of sympotms is the key-note of homoeopathy.

A pathologist examines a sick person from head to foot and finds no proof of sickness. And still the person under examination complains that he has a long list of sufferings. He has no refreshing sleep, has aches and pains, and various discomforts, always perplexed, worried and uneasy.

Homoeopathy reads these symptoms which are the language of nature and indicate and focus the internal sickness leading to some major disaster.

The stage of clear diagnosis comes when the breakdown occurs, the vital force gives way and you have consumption, fatty degeneration of heart or cirrhosis of liver and so on.

One has to agree that the patient is sick before the localisation of the diseases.

Dr. J.T. Kent observes, "Under traditional methods, it is necessary that a diagnosis be made before the treatment can be settled, but in most cases, the diagnosis cannot be made until results of the disease have rendered the patient incurable."

So we need to study the internal and the external man separately. The man feels, sees, tastes, bears, thinks and lives as also he wills and understands. The body is the house where the internal man resides. To illustrate, Dr. James Tyler Kent says, "One who is suffering from conscience, does not need a surgeon, but a priest. He who has a lacerated wound, or a broken bone or deformities, has need of a surgeon. If his tooth must come out, he must have a surgeon dentist.

If the physician acts also as a surgeon, he should stiches up a wound, but should not burn out an ulcer with nitrate of silver."

When "signs and symptoms are present the physician is needed, because these come from interior to exterior."

Our aim should be to discriminate and remove the external causes and turn into order, internal disorders.

For example, a comes to us with a bad food habit and if we keep on giving him Nux vomica, it is not advisable.

"Vicious habits, bad living, living in dampness are externals and must be removed. When a man avoids these externals, is clearly, carefully chooses his food, and has a comfortable home, **and is still miserable,** he must be treated from within."

A physician has to strengthen the vital force, increase

resistence, decrease the susceptibility and allow the nature to heal the patient perfectly and soundly.

There are wrong notions that homoeopathy is not very quick, it is not suitable for all occasions, it is useful as a palliative and that it requires a long time to cure. It is not so, not at all so.

The disappointments occur only when we are out of the track. A homoeopath seeks to establish a harmony and co-incidence between the language of ailments and the language of drug action. He has to be conscious of the drug properties with regard to their reaction on a healthy body in all aspects, i.e. physical and mental which include feelings, sensations, cravings, aversions, ameliorations, aggravations, time, weather conditions, temperaments etc. etc. Both the similars—when meet together, neutralise the disease conditions, and at the same time help the resistence to increase its power against susceptibility to disease forces.

In practice, we find sometime, such situations when either the symptoms are not so very clear in their indications or if they are clear, the durgs do not react. Our masters have covered most of such situations with directions to handle them. But these require to be arranged and illustrated in full context to be made more useful to the people and profession. This shall be the subject matter of subsequent volumes.

Dr. K.D. Kanodia

A-213 Kewal Park
Azadpur, Delhi-33

1. WORDS OF INSPIRATION

"One consults and quotes from several of our prescribing **geniuses** because one man has more completely grasped the inwardness and has had more **experience with one remedy,** another with another. For the same reason, it is well to read and study the same durg in several books to get enlightment always from the man best qualified to enlighten. Pick plenty of brains if you want to nourish and stimulate your own."

Dr. M.L. Tyler

"Homoeopathy, properly understood, offers a distinct contribution to medicine, and it has been narrow conception of what constitutes the healing art that has excluded it from the general profession. That of itself it has fallen into the hands of the incompetent and unscrupulous is no excuse for failing to investigate its actual merits. If the science of medicine is to be restricted to its own discoveries it is doomed."

Dr. C.M. Boger

"We not only need, but must have homoeopathic literature of a higher grade to interpret our art in an appealing, intelligent concise, and convincing manner to the intelligent mind."

Dr. Arthur B. Green

"The physician who fails to correct and simplify the diet in harmony with good sense is unintentionally having serious obstacles to recovery unremoved and to that extent he is falling short of the physician's highest and the only calling (which) is to restore health to the sick."

Dr. Underhill

2. WONDERS OF A SINGLE DOSE

ARNICA: I have come to the conclusion that in every case after the delivery, absolutely in every case, I have to give a dose of Arnica, I have never had the slightest trouble in many cases, because I always have Arnica, and in abortions after the abortion, always Arnica, and there is always something more to come, and it comes out easily and everything is safe, and absolutely no lesion.

Dr. F.K. Bellokossy

ANTIM TART: It has the nausea, vomiting, loose stools, prostration, cold sweat, and stupor or drowsiness found in almost all bad cases of this disease, and I have seldom been obliged to give more than two or three doses, one after each vomiting before the case was relieved.

Dr. E.B. Nash

ARSENICUM ALBUM: I remember a case of asthma of years' standing to which I was called at midnight, because they were afraid the patient would die before morning. Found that her attacks always come on at 1 A.M. Gave Arsenicum alb. 30th, and she was completely cured by it.

Dr. E.B. Nash

ARNICA: I have seen a sprained ankle when it was black and blue, so swollen that the shoe could not be put on, but after a dose of Arnica, the swelling disappeared in an astonishing way, the discolouration faded out and the patient was able to stand on the foot.

Dr. J.T. Kent

AURUM MUR NATRONATUM: While on a visit to New York city, I called upon Dr. M. Baruch, partly to see the man who had been reported time as both very skillful as a prescriber and eccentric as a man. During my call I stated to him my case. He prescribed for me a dose of Aurum muriaticum natronatum 1000th, followed by a powder each of Veronica officinalis 500th, 200th and 30th, and directed me to take them in the order named once in sixty hours and said: "In three months you will be well." I took the powders as directed and have never been troubled in that way since.

Dr. E.B. Nash

ALOE: I was called to treat a child five years of age suffering from birth with a most obstinate form of constipation. He had to be forced and held to the stool crying and screaming all the while being totally unable to pass any faeces even after an enema. I then gave a few doses of Aloe 200th and cured the whole trouble quickly and permanently.

Dr. E.B. Nash

BELLADONNA: The elder Lippe once told me of a case of suspicious enlargement or swelling and pain of the breast of long standing, which, as he expressed it, seemed likely to prove a case for the surgeon (cancer), which was entirely cured by a few doses of Belladonna, to which he was guided by this symptom of the pains being so much worse on lying down. Since then I have observed and verified this symptom in many cases of different kinds. I will not stop to give all the symptoms that might be present in Belladonna headaches.

Dr. E.B. Nash

CADMIUM: I frequently find cancer of the liver yielding to Calcarea ars. in every way but with the tendency to relapse, when a single dose of Cadmium in high potency will render the cure permanent.

Dr. A.H. Grimmer

HINA: After profuse bleeding in delivery, a dose of China M, dilution will recoup the strength of the patient.

Dr. R.B. Das

AUSTICUM: I was once called, in consultation, to a case f prosopalgia which had for a long time baffled the skill of very good homoeopathic practitioner. Not being able to elieve the case, he had become demoralized, and as the pain nd suffering were very great he had resorted to anodynes, ut with the usual result of making the patient worse, after ne anodynes had worn out, then she was before. On looking ver the case carefully, I found in addition to the emaciated nd greatly debilitated condition of the patient, after so long uffering, that the pains came in paroxysms, that they were f a drawing nature, and that she had suffered from eczema or years, at different times, before this pain appeared. ulphur had been given, but without relief. So I advised ʼausticum. It was given, in the 200th, and a rapid and a ermanent cure was the result.

Dr. E.B. Nash

CHAMOMILLA: Dr. Tyrell said once to me: ''When the usband complains of the wife's being cross and irritable, nd he cannot get along with her, give him a dose of hamomilla and it has worked. I have done it many times.

Dr. Edwards

CALCAREA-CARB: It is astonishing that one single dose of he potency suitable to meet the state of disorder will make hat infant commence to digest its food, and appropriate from ts food the lime substance that it needs in its bones, and wherever else it needs it. All at once the teeth begin to grow;

the bones begin to grow; and the legs get stiff enough for him to begin to walk; and they will hold him up. It is astonishing what changes will take place under the various medicines that are suitable for the disturbances of the hair, the bones and nails.

Dr. J.T. Kent

COLCHICUM: The smell of food cooking nauseates to faintness. To illustrate the value of this symptom I will give a case of my own practice; it was also my first experience with a potency as high as the 200th. Patient was a lady, seventy-five years of age, who was suddenly seized with sickness at the stomach and vomiting of blood in large quantities; then bloody stools followed, which were at first profuse, then became small and of bloody mucus. There was great tenesmus and pain in the bowels. She had become so weak that she could not lift her head from the pillow. By actual count the number of stools passed on cloths in the bed was sixty-five, in twenty-four hours, the pains, number of passages and all symptoms were aggravated from sundown to sunrise.

Dr. E.B. Nash

Arsenic. Alb.: One of the worst cases of sciatica I never saw was cured with Arsenicum album, on the indications, worse at midnight, especially from 1 to 3 o'clock; burning pains; and the only temporary relief during the paroxysms, was from bags of hot, dry salt applied to the painful part.

The lady was a sister of Charles Saunders, of New York, of school reader fame, who was himself a cripple from allopathically treated sciatica. She, after suffering indescribable agony for six weeks, was cured rapidly and permanently with a dose of Jenichen's 8m. of Arsenicum album. So we see again that no remedy and no particular set of remedies can be entirely relied upon, but the indicated one can.

Dr. E.B. Nash

GRAPHITES: If you know a woman who is suffering from an old scar that has formed a lump, when she is about to go into confinement, give a dose of Graphites as a general remedy, unless some other special remedy is called for.

Dr. J.T. Kent

GRAPHITES: I once treated a case of eczema of the legs which was of twenty years' standing. It was in an old obese woman, and, by the way, that is the kind of subject in which this remedy is found most efficacious.

I gave her, on account of much burning of the feet, a dose of Sulphur cm. In two or three weeks an eruption was developed all over the body which exuded a glutinous, sticky fluid. One dose of Graphites cm., dry on the tongue, cured this as well as the eczema of the legs and left her skin as smooth as that of a child.

Dr. E.B. Nash

GRAPHITES: A child three years of age had eczema captitis. Under allopathic local treatment the eczema disappeared; but soon enterocolitis of a very obstinate character set in. Then the regulars could not "do" that as they had the eczema, and after they had given up the case, pronouncing it consumption of the bowels, the homoeopath (myself) was called in on the ground that he could do no harm if he could do no good (as they said).

Case — Child greatly emaciated, little or no appetite, very restless, and "stools brown fluid mixed with undigested substances, and of an intolerably foetid odor." Taking into the account the history of the suppressed eczema I prescribed Graphites 6m. (Jenichen) and in a short time a perfect cure was the result.

Dr. E.B. Nash

HYDROCEPHALUS: Give Hedera helix one drop one dose only. Next morning clear flow of fluid through the nose will appear and only one dose will cure. Give second dose if recurrence is threatended.

Dr. R. B. Dass

IRIS: I once had a case of stomach trouble in a middle-aged lady. She had frequent attacks of vomiting of a stringly, glairy mucus which was ropy, would hang in strings from her mouth to the receptacle on the floor. Then the substance vomited became dark-coloured; like coffee grounds. She became very weak, vomited all nourishment. She also had profuse secretion of ropy saliva.

Thinking she had cancer of the stomach, she made her will and set her house in order, to die. Kali bichromicum was given with no benefit whatever, but Irish cured her completely in a short time and she remains well ten years since.

Dr. E.B. Nash

IODIUM: I have cured many cases of goitre with Iodine cm., every night for four nights, after the moon fulled and was waning.

Dr. E.B. Nash

KALI-CARBONICUM: The father-in-law of Dr. T.L. Brown,

an anaemic old man, was apparently near his end with hydrothorax and general dropsy. Dr. Brown was a skillful prescriber, but in this case had utterly failed to even relieve. In consultation with Dr. Sioan, after carefully reviewing the case, the fact appeared through the daughter of the patient, who had been his nurse all the time, that all his symptoms were aggravated at 3 A.M. Now Kali carb. 200 was given, and with such miraculous results that in an incredibly short time the old man was well and never had a return of that trouble. He lived for several years after, and, finally, did not die of dropsy at all.

Dr. E.B. Nash

KALI-IOD: A single dose of a very high potency of Kali iod. will turn things into order in persons subject to these hives and they will not come again.

Dr. J.T. Kent

LECHESIS: In many cases its action of one dose not only lasts for several days, weeks and months but sometimes one or two doses of Lachesis have cured the very chronic and the most complicated cases for ever.

Dr. B. Prasad Gupta

LYCOPODIUM: It is one of our best remedies for impotence. (Agnus castus). An old man marries his second or third wife and finds himself not "equal to the occasion." It is very embarassing for the whole family. A dose of Lycopodium sets the thing all right and makes the doctor a warm friend on both sides of the house.

Young men from onanism or sexual excess become impotent. The penis becomes small, cold and relaxed. The desire is as strong as ever, and perhaps more so, but he can't perform. (Selenium, Caladium). I have known apparently hopeless cases of this kind cured by the use of this remedy, high single doses at intervals of a week or more. Give it low, however, if you want to, but do not blame me if you don't succeed.

Dr. E.B. Nash

LACHESIS: Headache extending into nose, comes mostly in acute catarrh, especially when the discharge has been suppressed or stops after sleep. This kind of headache is often found in hay fever, with frequent and violent paroxysms of sneezing. Now if the hay fever paroxysms of a sneezing are decidedly worse after sleeping, even in the day time, Lachesis 200th may stop the whole business for the season.

Dr. E.B. Nash

LACHESIS: I once had a case of very obstinate constipation in an old syphilitic case. He was at last taken with very severe attacks of colic. The pains seemed to extend all through the abdomen, and always came on at night. After trying various remedies until I was discouraged, for he "got no better fast," he let drop this expression, "Doctor, if I could only keep awake all the time, I would never have another attack." I looked askance at him. "I mean," said he, "that I sleep into the attack, and waken in it." I left a dose of Lachesis 200. He never had another attack of the pain, and his bowels become perfectly regular from that day and remained so.

Dr. E.B. Nash

LACHESIS: In chronic cases wait patiently and see its deep and intense action. I have seen its working of one dose of thirty potency for months. One dose of thirty dilution has cured in my hands not only one case but patients after patients. In one case, dyspnoea with heart palpitation, severe and intolerable pains of left side before menses, blackish menses, falling of hair, over-sensitive to light etc., all these symptoms were of several years one dose of thirty potency cured.

Dr. B. Prasad Gupta

MAGNESIA-CARB: I once cured a severe case of coccydynia, a case of long standing. The pains were sudden, piercing, causing the patient to almost faint away. Magnesia carb. 200 cured promptly.

Dr. E.B. Nash

MERCURIUS: The chill is peculiar as I have observed it. It is not a shaking chill, but is simply creeping chilliness. Often when this creeping chilliness is felt it is the first symptom of a cold that has been taken, and, if left alone, the coryza, sore throat, bronchitis or even pneumonia may follow; but, if taken early, a dose of Mercurius may prevent all such troubles. The chilliness is felt most generally in the evening and increases into the night if not removed by Mercury. It also alternates with flashes of heat; first chilly, then hot, then chilly, etc., like Arsenicum. It is often felt in single parts. Then again it is felt in abscesses and is the harbinger of pus formation. If pus has already formed, especially much of it, the only thing Mercury can do is to hasten its discharge; but if little or none is actually formed a dose of Mercury high will often check the formation and a profuse sweat often follows with a subsidence of the swelling and a rapid cure of the disease.

Dr. E.B. Nash

MERCURIUS: If anyone is skeptical as to the efficiency of the very high potencies, I invite him to a test in just such a case. Give a single dose, dry upon the tongue or if you must seem to do more, dissolve a powder in four tablespoonfuls of water and give in half-hourly doses. Then wait, I have done it many times and an convinced.

Dr. E.B. Nash

NATRUM MUR: I have seen a patient who had lost 40 pounds of flesh (weight, 160 1b.), though eating well all of the time, under one dose of Natrum mur., tip the scales at 200 1bs. within three months from the time of taking, he was very hypochondriac at the time of the beginning of treatment.

Dr. E.B. Nash

NUX VOMICA: Inefficient labour pains, extending to rectum, with desire for stool or frequent urination, are quickly relieved, and become efficient, after the administration of a dose of Nux vomica 200.

Dr. E.B. Nash

PSORINUM: It is also found useful in the consequences of suppressed eruptions, and in such cases should never be forgotten when other anti-psorics fail. Dr. Wm. A. Hawley, of Syracuse, N.Y., once made a brilliant cure of a very bad case of dropsy in an old woman, being led to prescribe this remedy by the apperance of the skin. One dose of Fincke's 42m. potency, dry on the tongue, cured the whole case in a very short time.

Dr. E.B. Nash

PETROLEUM: I have cured a case of eczema of the lower

legs of twenty years' standing, always worse in winter, with one prescription of the 200th. I have cured chapped hands the same way. I once had a very obstinate case of chronic diarrhoea, but as soon as the fact that he had eczema of the hands in winter came to light I cured him quickly of the whole trouble with Petroleum 200.

Dr. E.B. Nash

PLUMBUM METALLICUM: I cured one case of post diphtheritic paralysis with it. It was a very severe case in a middle-aged man. His lower limbs were entirely paralyzed, and there was at the same time a symptom which I never met before, nor have I since, in such a case, viz., excessive hyperaesthesia of the skin. He could not bear to be touched anywhere, it hurt him so. After much hunting I found this hyperaesthesia perfectly pictured in Allen's Encyclopaedia, and that, taken together with the paralysis, seemed to me good reason for prescribing Plumbum, which I did in one dose of Fincke's 40m., with the result of bringing about rapid and continuous improvement until a perfect cure was reached. He took only the one dose, for a repetition was not necessary.

Dr. E.B. Nash

PLUMBUM METALLICUM: The father-in-law of Dr. T.L. Brown, over seventy years of age, was attacked with a severe pain in the abdomen. Finally, a large, hard swelling developed in the kileocaecal region very sensitive to contact or to the least motion. It began to assume a bluish colour, and on account of his age and extreme weakness it was thought that he must die. His daughter, however, studied up the case, and found in Raue's Pathology the indications for Plumbum as given in therapeutic hints for typhlitis. It was administered in the 200th potency, which was followed by relief and perfect recovery.

Dr. E.B. Nash

STICTA PULMONARIA: When after a wound, sprain or fracture, the patient tells you, "Since my accident, I do not have sound sleep. I sleep badly; one dose of Sticta pulmonaria 200 brings sleep. This is a remedy with the characteristic that it does not habitually work on insomnia, but it makes the fracture victim sleep.

Dr. Pierre Schmidt

STAPHISAGRIA: In one case, with the 200th of this remedy, I removed an excrescence on the perineum of a lady in which the growth was an inch long and the appearance was exactly in appearance like cauliflower. It rapidly disappeared under the action of this remedy and never returned.

Dr. E.B. Nash

SYPHILINUM: It has cured spasmodic bronchial asthma of twenty-five years standing.

Dr. B. Prasad Gupta

SILICEA: I have several times found a Silicea child suffering from epileptiform spasms which were always worse at new moon. A few doses of Silicea 200 set them all right.

Dr. E.B. Nash

TUBERCULINUM: Dr. Swan cured a case of headache of forty-five years' standing with Tuberculinum.

Dr. B. Prasad Gupta

TUBERCULINUM: One case of retarded menstruation in a young girl who had greatly enlarged tonsils and who began to grow tired and weak, pale and short breathed on any exercise. The menses appeared twice under the action of Pulsatilla, but at intervals of several other remedies to give her any benefit, she took one dose of Tuberculinum 1m. with prompt, easy and natural appearance of the menses and corresponding improvement in other respects, and is now attending school in apparent good health.

Dr. E.B. Nash

TUBERCULINUM: A case of lung trouble brought to me over a year ago from Seneca Falls, N.Y., had been under allopathic treatment for four years and had been every summer up in the Adirondacks at Saranac, at a sanitarium established by Dr. Loomis, of New York, lung specialist. She continued to grow worse until I took her case in hand. Under the action of 2 doses of Sulphur cm. followed by Tuberc. cm. she is so improved that I think it would be hard to convince any one that she ever suffered from such conditions.

Dr. E.B. Nash

3. 'SHEET ANCHOR' IN
EMERGENCIES

ARNICA TINCTURE: Applied neat to a wasp or bee sting is wonderfully effective.

Dr. M. Blakey

CALCAREA CARB: When given in repeated dose of 30th dilution relieves the pain attending the biliary passage.

Dr. Hughes

COLOCYNTH: No remedy produces more severe colic than this one, and no remedy cures more promptly.

Dr. E.B. Nash

HYPERICUM: Quite supercedes the use of morphis after operations in my hand.

Dr. Helmuth

Nothing equals Hypericum in cases of masned fingers.

Dr. E.A. Farrington

MYRISTICA 3x: Called the homoeopathic knife, is almost specific drug to break open carbuncle.

Dr. W. Karo

MYRISTICA: Often does away with the use of knife. Acts more powerfully than any other remedy in this.

Dr. C.C. Boericke

MURIATIC ACID: Is useful in the last stage of dropsy from cirrhosis of liver.

Dr. E. A. Farrington

NATRUM MUR: Is one of our best remedies for chronic headaches.

Dr. E.B. Nash

Fracture of hand and finger bones: These knit more quickly with Symphytum 30 two or three times a day for a week.

Dr. Pierre Schmidt

STRAMONIUM: Is most important when pain is almost inbearable, driving to despair. It ameliorates at once, and hastens benign suppuration.

Dr. C.G. Raue

In the few cases of pericarditis, I have treated, Spigelia has done all that medicine could do.

Dr. Russell

4. QUICKEST PALLIATION POSSIBLE

ARNICA: Given immediately in fractures and dislocations, relieves the nervousness and pain like magic, both externally and internally.

Dr. R. Patel & Dr. Elias

ACONITE: If dysentery sets in with viol fever, Aconite in many cases cures the whole disease in 2 or 3 days.

Dr. Jahr

ANTIMONIUM SULPH. NIGR: It relieves itching of skin which frequently occurs in old people.

Dr. Rudolph F. Rabe

ARNICA: If given at once after a fracture, it almost instantly relieves the muscular spasms which often occur and relieves the shock.

Dr. Stearns

ANTIMONIUM CRUD: It is especially to be considered if the gastric derangement is of recent date. The process of digestion is hardly under way; the eructations taste of the food as he ate it, and the sufferer feels as if he must "throw up" before there will be any relief. In such a case a few pellets of Antimonium crudum on the tongue will often settle the business, save the loss of a meal, and all further suffering.

Dr. E.B. Nash

ARNICA will quiet the startings of fractured limb.

Dr. Hughes

ARNICA MONT: It is very beneficial not only in injuries

caused by severe contusions and lacerations of fibres, but also in the most severe wounds by bullets and blunt weapons; in the pains and other ailments consequent on extracting the teeth and other surgical operations whereby sensitive parts have been violently stretches; as also after dislocations of joints, after setting fractures of bones etc.

Dr. Samuel Hahnemann

CAUSTICUM: It is the routine remedy for retention of urine after operation.

Dr. D.M. Foubister

CHOLESTERINUM: It is specific for gall stone colic; relieves the distress at once.

Dr. Swan

CHAMOMILLA will stop vomiting of Morphia in a few minutes.

Dr. J.K. Kent

CANTHARIS 200 given internally quickly cures the inflamed and horrible swelling that may follow great bites.

Dr. M.L. Tyler

CAUSTICUM: In 6th dilution will give immediate relief to pain in cases of burns and scalds.

Dr. R.B. Das

COLOCYNTHIS: If I was disposed to be skeptical as to the power of the small dose to cure, Colocynthis would convince me, for I have so promptly cured severe colic in many cases, from a child to adults, and even in horses. Of course, every true homoeopath can respond a man to that.

Dr. T.L. Brown

CALCAREA SULPHURICA: I once had a case in which there was great pain in the region of the kidneys for a day and night. Then there was a great discharge of pus in the urine, which continued several days and weakened the patient very fast. A Chicago specialist had examined the urine a short time before, and had pronounced the case Bright's disease. I finally prescribed Calcarea sulphurica 12 and under its action she immediately improved and made a very rapid and permanent recovery.

Dr. E.B. Nash

CINA: I once had, at one time, and in one family, five cases of typhoid fever, and they were all very sick. There was no mistake about the diagnosis, and I speak thus positively, because some think that a child under the age of six years cannot have this disease. This child, five years of age, was the last one of the family attacked with the disease, and it pursued the same course as the others in its regular rise and fall of temperature, bloating of a abdomen, diarrhoea and other symptoms common to this disease. I resolved to give a few doses of Cina anyway, and to my surprise I found my patient much better every way at my next visit and the improvement progressed right along to complete recovery. I learned for good, that, for purposes of prescribing, the name of the disease was little account.

Dr. E.B. Nash

HAMAMELIS: In varicose veins of the leg, you will be delighted with the way in which the first or second dilution of Hamamelis will cure the pain.

Dr. Hughes

DIGITALIS PURPUREA: One day I saw an old but very strong man staggering across the road toward my office. I thought he was drunk, but on closer observation I noticed that his face looked purple, his lips bluish, and I stepped out and helped him in. He sat down and could not for a few minutes speak a word, but sat and struggled for breath. His pulse was very irregular and intermittent. He had been obliged to give up all manual labour and dared not go away from home on his business, that of bridge builder. Said he expected to die with this heart disease. I gave him Digitalis 2, a few drops in water. in a few days I saw him shoveling snow from the walk in front of his dwelling. "Hello," he said, "I have no heart disease;" and I saw him often after that and he told me that that medicine cured him of those spells."

Dr. E.B. Nash

PULSATILLA: Pulsatilla will very often cause in five minutes a very strong contraction of the uterus, sometimes almost in a painless way.

Dr. J.T. Kent

LAPIS ALBUS: I put her upon Lapis albus as an experiment, for I had no hope she could live more than two weeks at the longest. Under the action of this remedy she began to improve immediately, and from the half dead wreck that could not turn in bed without help, a skeleton, white as a ghost, she has steadily improved until she is now doing her own housework, the discharges having all ceased except her natural menses at her regular periods. The tumor grows smaller, and it seems as though she might get well. She takes a dose of Lapis albus 30th once a week.

Dr. E.B. Nash

PLANTAGO: Toothache with the 2x dilution of Plantago, will cure seven-tenths of all cases of this kind in about 15 minutes

Dr. Ruetlinger

PICRIC ACID: I found this remedy very useful in apparent failure of brain power in an old man who had always been strong up to within a year or so of the time he called on me He complained of heaviness in the occiput and inability to exert the mind to talk or think, and general tired "played-out" feeling. I feared brain softening but I gave him Picric acid 6th trit. and it promptly cured him.

Dr. E.B. Nash

RHUS TOX is the homoeopathic knife in appendicitis.

Dr. Biegler

RHUS TOX is beneficial to control the threatened Iritis and formation of pus.

Dr. Dewey

STAPHISAGRIA: It is required when an abdominal or other operation wound is unduly painful for no obvious reason

Dr. D.M. Foubister

HYOSCYAMUS is one of our best remedies for hiccough occurring after operations of the abdomen.

Dr. E.A. Farrington

SECALE CORNUTUM: All the toes were attacked with dry gangrene. A few doses of Secale (high) afforded great relief, and checked the progress or the disease for a long time.

Dr. E.B. Nash

TARENTULA CUBENSIS: I have seen felons which had kept patients awake night after night walking the floor in agony from the terrible pains so relieved in a very short time that they could sleep in perfect comfort until the swellings spontaneously discharged, and progressed to a rapid cure.

Dr. E.B. Nash

THUJA OCCIDENTALIS: For instance, a case of enuresis had resisted many seemingly indicated remedies, until the hands were discovered to be covered with warts, when a few drops of Thuja cured.

Dr. E.B. Nash

VIBERNUM Q: Cramps in the abdomen and legs of pregnant women are controlled very quickly by this remedy.

Dr. Hale

5. MIRACLE CURES IN DIFFICULT, CHRONIC AND INCURABLE CASES

ARGENTUM NITRICUM: It has cured prolonged and most inveterate ulceration of the stomach, when there has been vomiting of blood.

Dr. J.T. Ken

ANTIMONIUM CRUDUM: There is a form of diarrhoea which alternates with constipation, oftenest found with old people, where Antimonium crudum is the only remedy. Then it is also one of the best remedies for mucous piles; there is a continuous oozing of mucus staining the linen, very disagreeable to the patient.

Dr. E.B. Nash

AMMONIUM CARB: It has cured the cough of Influenza when every thing else has failed, and I have more than once not found it necessary to give a second dose.

Dr. Youna

ARGENTUM NITRICUM: In dull chronic headaches of literary and businessman, Argentum nitricum is much commended.

Dr. Hughe

ANTIMONIUM CRUDUM: Some of the worst cases of chronic rheumatism have been cured by this remedy, guided by the excessive tenderness of the soles of the feet.

Dr. E.B. Nash

APIS MELLIFICA: Sensation as if every breath would be his last is very characteristic, and occurs not only in dropsical troubles of the chest, but seems also to be a nervous symptom.

Dr. E.B. Nash

ARNICA: I have come to the conclusion that in every case after the delivery, absolutely in every case, I have to give a dose of Arnica, I have never had the slightest trouble in many cases, because I always have Arnica, and in abortions after the abortion, always Arnica, and there is always something more to come, and it comes out easily and everything is safe, and absolutely no lesion.

Dr. F.K. Bellocossy

ARGENTUM MET: You will be astonished to know that homoeopathic remedies are wonderful in their ability to create tonicity, and thereby restore the prolapsed uterus to its normal position, and to remove the dragging down feeling women generally describe, a sensation as if the inner parts were being forced out.

Dr. J. T. Kent

APIS MELLIFICA: A number of years ago I was called to Watkins Glen, N. Y., in consultation in a very bad case of diptheria. One had already died in the family and four lay dead in the place that day. Over forty cases had died in the place and there was an **exodus** going on for fair. Her attending physician, a noble, whitehaired old man, and withal a good and able man, said, when I looked up to him and remarked I was rather young to counsel him; "Doctor, I am on my knees to anybody, for every case has died that has been attacked." The patient was two rooms away from us, but I could hear her difficult breathing even then. Apis was comparatively a new remedy then for that disease, but as I looked into her throat I saw Apis in a moment, and a few questions confirmed it. I told the doctor what I thought and asked him if he had tried it. He said, no, he had not thought of it, but it was a powerful blood poison; try it. It cured the case, and not one case that took this remedy from the beginning, and persistently, died. It was the remedy for the genus epidemicus.

Dr. E. B. Nash

ANACARDIUM ORIENTALE: In the fall of 1899 I was called to a lady, married, 35 years of age, mother of three children.

She was quite emaciated, with a yellowish cachectic look of the face. A couple of years before I treated her when she had an attack of vomiting, in which she vomited coffee-ground substances.

She was relieved at that time by a dose of Arsenicum alb. 40m., but had more or less trouble with her digestion up to this time. This last attack was more persistent and did not yield to Arsenicum and some other remedies.

After a while it appeared that the pain (which was very severe) and vomiting came on when the stomach was empty. She had to eat once or twice in the night for relief. The substance vomited was always black or brown looking like coffee-grounds. Her sister had been operated for cancer of the breast, and of course she was very nervous and fearful of cancer of the stomach, Anacardium relieved promptly, and she has had no return of the trouble since then.

Dr. E. B. Nash

ARNICA: I once cured a man who had suffered from what

he and his physician had called dyspepsia for several years. He had been obliged to give up his business because he could not eat enough to support his strength. He had been told by his physician that he would never be well again and had given up hopes himself. This condition was caused by the kick of a horse upon the region of the stomach. A few doses of Arnica 200 cured him in a short time and he resumed his business.

Dr. E. B. Nash

BORAX: The ears discharge. I cured a case of otorrhoea of fourteen years' standing with this remedy.

Dr. E. B. Nash

COLLINSONIA: With Collinsonia I once cured a very severe colic which had been of frequent occurrence in a lady for several years and had completely baffled the old school efforts to cure. I was led to choose the remedy on account of the obstinate constipation, the great flatulence and the haemorrhoidal condition present.

Dr. E. B. Nash

CAUSTICUM: This is like Nux vomica and Cantharis, and I once cured a chronic case of cystitis in a married woman, which had baffled the best efforts of several old school physicians, eminent for their skill, for years.

Dr. E. B. Nash

CONIUM: It is perhaps the first remedy to be thought of in all cases of tumors, scirrhous or otherwise, coming on after contusions, especially if they are of stony hardness and heavy feeling.

Dr. E. B. Nash

CHINA: It is one of the best remedies in chronic liver troubles. There is pain in the right hypochondria, and often the liver may be felt below the ribs, enlarged, hard and sensitive to touch.

Dr. E. B. Nash

CARBO ANIMALIS: It has relieved in incurable cases and has apparently removed the cancerous condition for years, even though it comes back afterwards and kills. This remedy is often a great palliative for the pains that occur in cancer, the indurations and the stinging, burning pains.

Of course we do not want to teach, nor we wish to have you infer, that a patient with a well-advanced cancerous affection, such as scirrhus may be restored to perfect health, and the cancerous affection removed.

Any one who goes around boasting of the cancer cases has cured ought to be regarded with suspicion.

Dr. J. T. Kent

CISTUS: I remember the first time my attention was decidedly called to Cistus. I had put it on my list to study from time and have come to the conclusion that it was only a side issue, until a young lady, nineteen years of age fell under my observation. The glands of the neck were large and hard, the parotids especially she had foetid otorrhoea; her eyes were inflamed and suppurating; there were fissures at the corners of the eyes; her lips were cracked and bleeding, and she had salt rheum at the end of the fingers. I could not make Calcarea fit the patient but after much study this little remedy seemed to be just what I needed; and although she had an immense amount of homoeopathy, good and bad, this remedy cured.

Dr. J. T. Kent

CARBO VEGETABILIS: Vital forces nearly exhausted, cold surface, especially from knees down to feet; lies motionless, as if dead; breath cold; pulse intermittent, thready; cold sweat on limbs. This is truly desperate condition. Then add to these symptoms, blood stagnates in the capillaries, causing blueness, coldness and ecchymoses; the patient so weak he cannot breathe without being constantly fanned. Gaps: "Fan me: Fan me:" Carbo **veg.** has saved such cases.

Dr. E. B. Nash

CROTALUS HORRIDUS: It seems, so far, to have shown its greatest usefulness in diseases which result in a decomposition of the blood of such a character as to cause haemorrhages from every outlet of the body (Acetic acid); even the sweat is bloody.

Dr. E. B. Nash

CANTHARIS VESICATORIA: The mucus was so profuse, and tenacious, and ropy, that I thought of **Kali bichromicum,** and thought it must be the remedy; but it did not even ameliorate, and she got worse all the time, until one day she mentioned that she had great cutting and burning on urinating, which she must do very frequently.

On the strength of the urinary symptom, for I knew nothing of its curative powers on the respiratory organs at that time, I gave her **Cantharis.** The effect was magical.

It is needless to describe the mutual delight of both physician and patient in such a case, for it was astonishing the rapidity with which the perfect and permanent cure of the case was accomplished.

Dr. E. B. Nash

CANNABIS   SATIVA: It is the remedy par excellence with which to begin the treatment of gonorrhoea, unless some other remedy is particularly indicated, and such cases are very few. The most characteristic symptom is that the urethra is very sensitive to touch or external pressure. The patient cannot walk with his legs close together because any pressure along the tract hurts him so. If the diseases has extended up the urethra, or into the bladder, there will often be severe pains in the back every few minutes and the urine may be bloody. I used in my early practice to put five drops mother tincture into four ounces of water (in a four-ounce vial) and let the patient take a teaspoonful three times a day. After about four days the inflammatory symptoms would have subsided, and the thin discharge have thickened and become greenish in appearance.   Then Mercurius solubilis 3d tritura-tion, a powder three times a day, would often finish the case. Or if a little, thin, gleety discharge remained, I cured that with Sulphur, Capsicum or Kali iodide. I have cured many cases from one to two weeks this way. Later I have used the c.m potency in the first stage, and sometimes never have to use the second remedy. If I do Mercurius corrosivus c.m is generally the remedy. Sometimes Pulsatilla, Sulphur, or Sepia to finish up the case. There are exceptions, but the rule is that cases get well promptly under this treatment.

Dr. E. B. Nash

CHELIDONIUM MAJUS: Sometimes in coughs which are persistent with much pain through right side of chest and into shoulder, Chelidonium helps us out and saves the patient from what might easily terminate in consumption.

Dr. E. B. Nash

COLCHICUM AUTUMNALE: I had my Lippe text-book

of Materia Medica in my carriage and I went out and got it and sat down by the bedside; determined to find that peculiar and persistent symptom and "fight it out on that line if it took all summer." I had a box of Dunham's 200th under my carriage seat that had been there for over a year, but which I have never used for want of confidence in high potencies. It was the best I could do for the present, so I dissolved a few pellets in a half glass of cold water, and directed to give one teaspoonful after every passage of the bowels. On my way home I stopped my horse two or three times to turn around and go back and give that poor suffering woman some medicine. I felt guilty, but I said to myself this is Lippe's Materia Medica, and these are Carrol Dunham's potencies, and here is a clear cut indication for its administration, and the other symptoms do not counter-indicate. Well, I got home. But I started early the next morning to try and make amends for my rashness (if the patient was not dead) of yesterday. Imagine my surprise as I stepped into the sick-room when my patient slowly turned her head upon the pillow and said, with a smile, "Good morning, Doctor." I had been met with a groan several past mornings. I felt faint myself then. I dropped into a chair by the bedside and remarked, "You are feeling better." "Oh, yes, Doctor." "How much of that last medicine did you take?" "Two doses." "What!" "Two doses"; "I only had two more stools after you left." "Don't you have any more pain?" "Pain stopped like that" (putting her hands together) "and I feel well except weakness." She took no more medicine, quickly recovered, and was perfectly well for five years after.

Dr. E. B. Nash

CARBO VEGETABILIS: Chronic complaints following or dating back for years to some imperfectly cured of suppressed acute disease.

Dr. E. B. Nash

HELLEBORUS NIGER: These symptoms (head rolling from side to side on the pillow, with screams; great stupidity or soporous sleep; greedy drinking of water; wrinkled forehead with cold sweat; motion of jaws, as chewing something; continual motion of one arm and leg, while the other lies as if paralyzed; urine scanty or entirely suppressed, (sometimes sediment like coffee grounds) indicated a desperate condition, and the patient will soon die comatose or in convulsions unless the proper remedy can be found.

Helleborus niger can often cure such cases, as I have often observed, not only in my own practice, but in that of others. I have sometimes observed that the first sign of improvement in such cases was a decided increase in the urine, and following it a general subsidence of all the other bad symptoms. I have used it with most prompt and satisfactory results in the 1000th (B. & T.) and 33m, (Fincke's) potencies.

Dr. E. B. Nash

HYDRASTIS CANADENSIS: I have found it most efficacious in the 200th (B. & T.). I once cured a case that was of years' standing, had worn cathartics out, and all the way she could live (her words) was to swallow a spoonful of whole flax seed with every meal. I have used it in infantile constipation successfully, and it is most useful when all other symptoms aside from constipation are conspicuous for their absence.

Dr. E. B. Nash

KALI BICHROMICUM: Of course leucorrhoeas of both the

ropy and jelly-like variety come under this remedy and many
fine cures have resulted from its use.

Dr. E. B. Nash

KALI BICHROMICUM: I remember one case of years ago
in which such ulcers appeared in the throat of a woman. One
had eaten up through the soft palate into the posterior nares,
and the whole palate looked as though it would be destroyed
by the ulcerative process if not speedily checked. The case
had a syphilitic look to me and had been under the treatment
of two old school physicians for a long time. I gave Kali bich
30th, and to say that I was astonished at the effect (for it was
in my early practice) is putting it mildly, for the ulcers healed
so rapidly, and her general condition, which was very bad,
correspondingly improved, that in three weeks from that time
she was well to all appearance and never had any return of
the trouble afterwards, or for years, at least as long as I knew
her.

Dr. E. B. Nash

KALI HYDROIODICUM: 'Kali iod' in the words of E. A.
Farrington; "Pneumonia, in which disease it is an excellent
remedy when hepatization has commenced, when the disease
localizes itself, and infiltration begins. In such cases, in the
absence of other symptoms calling distinctively for Bryonia,
Phosphorus or Sulphur, I would advise you to select Iodine
or Iodide of Potassa. It is also called for when the nepatization
is so extensive that we have cerebral congestion, or even an
effusion into the brain as a result of this congestion.

Dr. E. B. Nash

KALI MURIATICUM: I have seen enlarged joints after
acute rheumatism repaidly reduced to normal size under its

action, sometimes after they had resisted other remedies a long time; but I do not know of any characteristic symptoms for its use in preference to other remedies.

Dr. E. B. Nash

KALI CARBONICUM: It has cured a number of cases of fibroid tumor long before it was time for the critical period to cure.

You must remember that there is a natural tendency for a fibroid to cease to grow at the climacteric period, and afterwards to shrivel and that this takes place without any treatment, but the appropriate remedies will cause that haemorrhage to cease, will cause that tumor to cease, to grow and after a few days there will be ground shrinkage in its size.

Dr. J. T. Kent

KALMIA LATIFOLIA: I remember a patient, an old syphilitic, who was told if he ever made a violent more he would die, the valves of his heart were so badly affected. He had all the murmurs that it seemed possible from the heart valves. He had travelled all over and had taken large doses of Mercury, and his syphilitic condition had to a great extent been suppressed, until finally the whole trouble had located in the heart. Kalmia removed all the dyspnoea and palpitation in a few months, and it was nearly two years before there was a marked return of the symptoms and a repetition put him in a state of health, so that he needed no more medicine. This shows that what a deep-acting remedy Kalmia is, how long it may act, what wonderful change it may effect. A remedy must be capable of going deep into the life to do such things.

Dr. J. T. Kent

KALI CARBONICUM: It is not only a great remedy for pneumonia, pleurisy and heart troubles, as there spoken of, but goes much further and becomes very useful in incipient and even with advanced cases of phthisis pulmonalis. I have seen a case pronounced incurable by several old experienced and skillful physicians, Dr. T. L. Brown among them, get well under a dose once in eight days of Kali carb.

Dr. E. B. Nash

MURIATIC ACID: It cures the muscular weakness following excessive use of opium and tobacco. (Veratrum alb., Puls., Avena-s., Ipec.)

Dr. H. C. Allen

MERCURIUS: It cures lingering febrile conditions analogous to the typhoid state, but caused by suppressed ear discharge. I have cured cases that were due to packing the ear with borax, idoform, etc., the patient having first a remittent and later a continued fever. This would go on for five or six weeks and be relieved only when the discharge returned after a dose of Merc. I remember a case of this type. It was called cerebrospinal meningitis; the head was drawn back and twisted and held to one side. It began as on otitis media with discharge which was suppressed. Two or three doctors were called and could do nothing. In the night I went to the bedside and got the history and symptoms of Mercurius. Merc. re-established the discharge in twenty-four hours, the torticollis passed away, the fever subsided and the child made an excellent recovery. I can recall many such cases.

Dr. J. T. Kent

MURIATIC ACID: It is useful in the last stage of Dropsy from cirrhosis of liver.

Dr. E. A. Farrington

LACHESIS: H. N. Guernsey: "If pus has already formed in ovaritis, Lachesis may be the most appropriate remedy to promote its escape externally or through the intestines."

Dr. B. Prasad Gupta

LACHESIS: In many chronic cases its action of one dose not only lasts for several days, weeks and months but sometimes one or two doses of Lachesis have cured the very chronic and the most complicated cases for ever.

Dr. B. Prasad Gupta

LYCOPODIUM: It has often saved neglected, mal-treated or imperfectly cured cases of pneumonia from running into consumption. It may even come into the later stages of the acute attack itself, and here as usual the disease is apt to be in the right lung, and especially if liver complications arise. The disease has passed the first or congestive stage, and generally the stage of hepatization, or is in the last part of this stage, and is trying hard to take a favourable turn into the breaking up of third stage, the stage of resolution. Just here is where many cases die, neither free expectoration, nor perfect absorption of the disease product taking place. There is extreme dyspnoea, the cough sounds as if the entire parenchyma of the lung were softened; even raising whole mouthfuls of mucus does not afford relief, the breath is short and the wings of the nose expand to their utmost with a fan-like motion. Now is the time when Lycopodium does wonders. Again, even when this stage is imperfectly passed, and the patient still coughs and expectorates much thick, yellow, purulent or greyish-yellow, purulent (sometimes foetid) matter, tasting salty, with much rattling in the chest, Lycopodium is indispensable.

Dr. E. B. Nash

LACHESIS: I once had a case of very obstinate constipation in an old syphilitic case. He was at last taken with very severe attacks of colic. The pains seemed to extend all through the abdomen, and always came on at night. After trying various remedies until I was discouraged, for he "got no better fast," he let drop this expression, "Doctor, if I could only keep awake all the time, I would never have another attack." I looked askance at him. "I mean," said he, "that I sleep into the attack, and waken in it." I left a dose of Lachesis 200. He never had another attack of the pain, and his bowels became perfectly regular from that day and remained so.

Dr. E. B. Nash

LAC CANINUM: Two cases of tonsillitis in one house in separate families, I was called to treat one of them, and a very excellent allopathic physician the other. Of course, there was close watching to see which case would get well the quickest, and especially if either could be cured without suppuration taking place. They were both very bad cases. Both progressed rapidly for forty-eight hours. In my case the swelling began on one side; the next day was even worse on the other side, so I told them that as the first side was better I thought the last one would be better tomorrow; but alas the next day number one was worse again, the patient could not swallow, food and drinks came back by the nose. It was with much difficulty, choking and struggling that even a spoonful of medicine could be taken. I hesitated no longer, but gave Lac caninum c.m. at noon, and when I visited her in the evening found her taking oyster broth and she could speak distinctly, whereas she could not articulate a word in the morning. In another day the patient was well expect some weakness.

Dr. E. B. Nash

LAC CAMINUM: It cured the case very quickly. Not long after I had a very severe case of scarlatina. The throat was swollen full, and the restlessness was so marked with pains in the limbs which left the patient tossing from side to side that I thought surely Rhus tox. must be the remedy. But it failed to relieve. Then I discovered that the soreness of the throat and the pains alternated sides. This called my mind to the remedy, which was given with prompt relief. I used the c.m. in this case.

Dr. E. B. Nash

NATRUM MURIATICUM: It affects a radical cure of constipation when many boasted and popular remedies fail. It is a regulator of water in the system and if moisture is drawn from rectum, loss of function results and produces constipation.

Dr. Heselton

PODOPHYLLUM: It is excellent in moderate attacks of jaundice without fever, in chronic jaundice not much interfering with the general health.

Dr. Hempel

PHOSPHORUS: In tuberculosis, it is oftenest indicated in the incipient stage with the symptom of cough, oppression and general weakness already mentioned; but I have often found it indicated in the later stages, and if given very high and in the single dose and not repeated have seen it greatly benefit even incurable cases. If given too low and repeated it will fearfully aggravate.

Dr. E. B. Nash

PLUMBUM: Some years ago a physician came to me in regard to his wife. She had been unconscious for two days and had passed no urine for days and the catheter showed there was none in the bladder. She had quite an array of symptoms but they were common symptoms. She had the slowness for days before, and complained of a sensation of continual pulling at the navel, as if a string were drawing it back to the spinal column, and then the coma came on. In the middle of the night this doctor came to me in great distress. He said she was pale as death and breathing slow. A single powder of Plumbum high was given, and she passed urine in a few hours, roused up and never had such an attack again.

Dr. J. T. Kent

SULPHUR: Your former remedy was well chosen and seemed to help the patient in a measure, but the case relapses, lingers or progresses slowly to perfect recovery. It is on account of a depression of the vital force, as Hahnemann would call it. It may be on account of psora or not. Now give a dose of Sulphur and let it act a few hours if in an acute case, or a number of days if chronic. Then you may return to your former remedy and get results which you could not before the Sulphur was given. It clears up the case and prevents its becoming chronic or a lingering unsatisfactory convalescence.

Dr. E. B. Nash

SALICEA: The child takes nourishment enough, but, whether vomited or retained, goes on emaciating and growing weaker and weaker until it dies of inanition, unless Silicea checks this process. Many such cases have I saved with this remedy and made them healthy childern.

Dr. E. B. Nash

SILICEA: It builds them up, and so it seems, for under its action the patient's spirits rise, hope revives, the weakness and depression give way to a feeling of returning strength and health. It makes no difference whether the ulcerations are in the tissues already named, in the lungs, intestinal tract, or mammae, or elsewhere, the effect is the same, and the improvement in the local affection generally follows the general constitutional improvements.

Dr. E. B. Nash

STRAMONIUM: One was a lady about thirty years of age, who was overheated in the sun, on an excursion. She was a member in good standing in the Presbyterian church, but imagined herself lost and called me in six mornings in succession to see her die. Lost, lost, lost, eternally lost, was her theme, begging minister, doctor and everybody to pray for, and with her. Talked night and day about it. I had to shut her up in her room alone for she would not sleep a wink or let anyone else.

She imagined her head was as big as a bushel and had me examine her legs, which she insisted were as large as a church. After treating her several weeks with Glonoine, Lach., Natrum carb. and other remedies on the cause as the basis of the prescription, without the least amelioration of her condition, I gave her Stramonium, which covered her symptoms, and in twenty-four hours every vertigo of that mania was gone. But for the encouragment I gave the husband that I could cure her she would have been sent to the Utica Asylum, where her friends had been advised to send her by the allopaths. I gave her the sixth dilution or potency.

Dr. E. B. Nash

STRAMONIUM: The whole inner mouth as if raw; the tongue after a while may become stiff or paralyzed. Stools loose, blackish, smelling like carrion, or no stool or urine. Later there may be complete loss of sight, hearing, and speech with dilated, immovable pupils and drenching sweat which brings no relief, and death must soon close the scene unless Stramonium helps them out.

Dr. E. B. Nash

STICTA PULMONARIA: I have relieved many cases of chronic catarrh with Sticta; some of years' standing.

Dr. E. B. Nash

SULPHUR: A lady (maiden) had been an invalid for fourteen years. Her trouble seemed to centre in her stomach. So that for all that long period of time she could eat nothing but a little Graham bread and milk, hardly enough to sustain life, and in the earlier part of her sickness for a long time was able only to take a teaspoonful of milk at a time. She was an almost literal walking skeleton. I found, after much questioning and several failures to relieve her much, that about fifteen years before she had with an ointment suppressed an eczema of the nape and occiput. She boasted that she had never seen a vertigo of it since. I gave that lady Sulphur 200 and in three weeks from that time had that eruption fully restored and her stomach trouble completely relieved.

Dr. E. B. Nash

SPIGELIA ANTHELUMINTICA: I treated in Gumpendorf Hospital at Viena, 57 cases of rheumatic carditis with but one death and Spigelia was the only medicine employed.

Dr. Fleishman

TUBERCULINUM: Dr. Swan cured a case of headache of forty-five years standing with Tuberculinum.

Dr. B. Prasad Gupta

TUBERCULINUM: In view of what Dr. Burnett has written, and my own limited experience lately, I am confident that Tuberculinum is destined to rank with Psorinum in the treatment of chronic diseases.

Dr. E. B. Nash

USTILAGO: Ustilago maydis has cured negro urticaria of six years standing.

Dr. B. Prasad Gupta

VERATRUM ALBUM: If we were to describe in one word the general condition, as near as possible, for which this remedy was best, it would be collapse. Let me quote: "Rapid sinking of forces; complete prostration; cold sweat and cold breath." "Skin blue, purple, cold, wrinkled, remaining in folds when pinched." "Face hippocratic; nose pointed." "Whole body icy cold." "Cold skin, face cold, back cold." "Hands icy cold." "Feet and legs icy cold." (Icy coldness of surface, covered with cold sweat, Tabacum.) "Cramps in calves." All these are verified symptoms, and show to what an extreme degree of collapse a case may come and yet be cured. This condition may be found in rapidly progressing, acute cases like cholera, or it may be found in suppressed exanthemata; or, again, in the course of bronchitis, pneumonia, typhoid or intermittent fever. No matter where found, or in connection with whatever disease, if this collapse is present, and especially if the grand keynote, "cold sweat on face and forehead," is present, we may give this remedy with full confidence that it will do all that can be done and much more than the old school system of stimulation with alcoholics.

Dr. E. B. Nash

ZINCUM METALLICUM: A young lady about 20 years of age complained, a week before I was called, of weakness, or feeling of general prostration; headache, and loss of appetite, but the greatest complaint was of prostration. She was a student and her mother, who was an excellent nurse, attributed all her sickness to overwork at school, and tried to rest and "nurse her up." But she continued to grow worse. I prescribed for her Gelsemium and followed it with Bryonia according to indications, and she ran through a mild course of two weeks longer, and seemed convalescing quite satisfactorily.

Being left in a room alone, while sleeping and perspiring, she threw off her clothes, caught cold and relapsed. Of course the "last stage of that patient was worse than the first." The bowels became enormously distended, profuse haemorrhage occurred, which was finally controlled by Alumen, a low form of delirium came on, the prostration became extreme notwithstanding the haemorrhage was checked, until the following picture obtained-staring eyes rolled upward into the head, head retracted; complete unconsciousness, lying on back and sliding down in bed, twitching, or rather intense, violent trembling all over, so that she shook the bed. I had nurses hold her hands night and day, she shook and trembled so; hippocratic face, extremities deathly cold to knees and elbows, pulse so weak and quick I could not count it, and intermittent; in short, all signs of impending paralysis of the brain. The case seemed hopeless, but I put ten drops of Zincum metallicum in two drams of cold water, and worked one-half of it between her set teeth, a little at a time, and an hour after the other half. About one hour after the last dose she turned her eyes down and faintly said, milk. Through a bent tube she swallowed a half glass of milk, the first nourishment she had received in 24 hours. She got no more medicine for four days, and improved steadily all the time. She afterward received a dose of Nux vomica and progressed rapidly to a perfect recovery. So Zincum 200 can, like other metals, perform miracles when indicated.

Dr. E. B. Nash

6. HOMOEOPATHY
VS.
ALLOPATHY

CROTON TIGLIUM: When the allopaths, in any case where they considered an operation of the bowels impera- tive, had exhausted all other resources, Croton tiglium was their "biggest gun for the last broadside." In other words, this is a most violent cathartic. Now if Similia, etc., is not true, Croton tig. ought utterly to fail to cure diarrhoea; but it is true, and notwithstanding this remedy has proved its truth over and over again the allopaths deny and reject homoe- opathy.

Dr. E. B. Nash

IPECACUANHA: I have cured many cases of fever and ague by the first prescription, thus saving myself a good deal of unnecessary seeking and comparing. Whatever may be said in condemnation of this loose prescribing, it is certainly preferable to the inevitable Quinine prescription of the old school, and some self-styled homoeopaths, for the reason that it will cure more cases than Quinine, and do infinitely less harm. Ipecac. can cure more cases than Quinine, but both can cure the case to which they are homoeopathic, and that in the potentized form of the drug. We have such clear-cut indi- cations for the use of many remedies that we need not fail once where the allopaths do twenty times, which their indis- criminate Quinine treatment.

Dr. Johr

OPIUM: This is the reason why the homoeopath can make his sleepless patient sleep a natural sleep with Opium in the little dose, while the allopath forces his patient into a stupor (not a sleep) with his big dose. The one is curative, the other poisonous.

Dr. E. B. Nash

PLATINA: I was led by it to prescribe the remedy in a very obstinate case of insanity which had resisted the skill of several allopathic physicians of note, and they had finally decided that the case must be sent to the insane asylum. The parents, however, who were quite wealthy, could not consent to that, and were induced to try homoeopathy. I gave her Platina on the strength of this mental indication, which was very prominent, coupled with another prominent symptom, which also appears under this remedy, viz., "physical symptoms disappear and mental symptoms appear," and vice versa. This physical symptom was a pain the whole length of the spine. This was the symptom alternating with the mental one. It was one of the most brilliant cures I ever saw. Improvement began the first day and never flagged, and she remained well now 15 years, with never a sign of return.

Dr. E. B. Nash

7. PATHOLOGY
AND
SYMPTOMATOLOGY

It must be remembered that chronic renal infection is an important cause of hypertension.

Dr. Kesava Pai

I consider Gelsemium 1x one of our best remedies for insomnia and there are no bad after effects.

Dr. Kuthbert

Immediately bathing with water as hot as can be borne for length of time, followed by a compress of Arnica, Aconite, Rhus tox. or Ruta. This treatment, employed promptly, generally cures at once.

Dr. Ruddock

Once of the most characteristic symptoms of the elaps provings is the marked aggravation from rain or the approach of rain, the aggravation from rain or its approach in elaps out generals this symptoms in Rhus tox.

Dr. H. A. Roberts

As regards laterality in Nux vomica abdominal symptoms find to be right sided, and chest symptoms left sided.

Dr. D. M. Gibson

There is scarcely a remedy that has much such marked symptoms of glossitis as Apis.

British Journal of Homoeopathy

Phosphorus although it has the marked symptom of

unquenchable thirst for cold drinks also is a thirstless remedy, a fact which is very easily overlooked.

Dr. Rudolph F. Rabe

I know some people who are made absolutely sleepless by Opium in all sorts of doses, and Opium 30 has helped me in cases of sleeplessness, as often as Coffea.

Dr. J. H. Clarke

It is essential to ascertain the seat of the local disease with accuracy; for, every experienced homoeopath knows how in toothache for instance, it is necessary to select the remedy which in its provings has repeatedly acted upon the very tooth that suffers.

The specific curative power of Sepia in those stubborn and sometimes fatal joint abscesses evidence upon this point, for they differ from similar gatherings in location only, while the remedies so suitable for abscess eslewhere remain ineffectual here.

Dr. C. M. Boger

What is the scirrhus but a peculiar form induration? When the economy takes on a low type of life, a low form of tissue making, and the tissues inflame and upon the slightest provocation indurate we can see that this is a kind of constitution that is predisposed to deep-seated troubles, to phthisis, Bright's disease, diabetes, cancer etc.

Dr. J. T. Kent

The cerebellum presides over respiration during sleep and the cerebrum presides over respiration when the patient is awake.

Dr. J. T. Kent

With every little trouble located in the heart there comes hopelessness, but when the mainfestation of disease is in the lungs there is hopefulness.

Dr. J. T. Kent

The first permanent and substantial indication that the remedy is working in a hydrocephaloid case is that it increases the flow of urine, which has been scanty all the time.

Dr. J. T. Kent

Do not be discouraged in prescribing if the pathological conditions do not go away; but if all the symptoms of the patient have gone away, and the patient is eating well, and is sleeping well, and doing well, do not feel that it is impossible for that opacity of the cornea to go away, for sometimes it will.

Dr. J. T. Kent

Woman who marries at 28 or 30, or later, suffer from prolonged labor.

Dr. J. T. Kent

BELLADONNA: Gurnesy says :— "That medicine is particularly applicable, and in fact takes the lead over all others in cases in which quickness or suddeness of either sensation or motion is predominant." To be sure all these symptoms have their pathological explanation if we could give it; but, acting on our law of Similia, we can cure our patients and are not left at sea, without chart or compass, becuase we cannot explain. We know that these symptoms are the natural outcry of the pathological state, and that the administration of a poison which is capable of setting up a similar outcry cures the patient.

Dr. E. B. Nash

I only tell you this to give you an idea how long it takes to restore order, for nature herself to replace the bad tissue and put healthy tissue in that same place, to restore an organ. It takes time, and it is best that we should not be surprised. It may be that the medicine has done all it can do. Here is another thing I have seen; even when there were no symptoms left, and after waiting a considerable time, there were no symptoms. I have seen another dose of the same medicine that was given on the last symptoms give the patient a great lift, and pathological conditions commence to go away. So Calcarea is a great friend to the oculist, and every physician ought to be just as good a prescriber as the oculist can be, for he prescribes for the patient. So must the oculist. In prescribing I am in doubt whether there can be any such thing as a speciality, because the homoeopathic physician prescribes for the patient. He prescribes for the patient, whether he has eye disease, ear disease, throat disease, lung disease, or liver disease, etc.

Dr. J. T. Kent

PODOPHYLLUM PELTATUM: All drugs have their double action, or what is called primary and secondary action. But the surest and most lasting curative action of any drug is that in which the condition to be cured simulates the primary action of the drug. For, as I have held elsewhere, I think that what is called secondary action is really not the legitimate action of the drug, but the aroused powers of the organism against the drug. So the alternate diarrhoea and constipation in disease is a fight, for instance, between the disease (diarrhoea) and the natural powers resisting it. It is of considerable importance then to be able to recognize in such a case whether it is the diarrhoea or constipation that is the disease, against which the alternate condition is the effort of the vital force to establish health. Yet such an understanding is not always absolutely imperative, for in either case there are generally enough concomitant symptoms to decide the choice of the remedy. Indeed, the choice must always rest upon either the peculiar and characteristic symptoms appearing in the case or the totality of them. None but the true homoeopathist learns to appreciate this. Here is, where what is called pathological prescribing often fails, for the choice of the remedy may depend upon symptoms entirely outside of the symptoms which go to make up the pathology of the case, at least so far as we as yet understand pathology.

Dr. E. B. Nash

PULSATILLA: It seems to me like folly to undertake to pose as either an exclusive pathologist or symptomatologist. Both pathology and symptomatology are valuable and inseparable; neither can be excluded. Pathology is what the doctor can tell (sometimes); symptomatology is what the patient can tell.

Dr. E. B. Nash

8. AGGRAVATIONS — WHICH ARE MEANINGFUL

CONIUM MACULATUM: I once treated a case of what seemed to be locomotor ataxia with this remedy.

The patient had been slowly losing the use of his legs; could not stand in the dark; and when he walked along the street would make his wife walk either ahead of him, or behind him, for the act of looking sidewise at her or in the least turning head or eyes that way would cause him to stagger or fall.

Conium cured him. I would always aggravate at first, but he would greatly improve after stopping the remedy. The aggravation was just as invariable after taking a dose of Fincke's cm. potency as from anything lower, but the improvement lasted longer after it.

Taking an occasional dose from a week to four weeks apart completely cured him in about a year. It was a bad case, of years' standing, before I took him.

Dr. E. B. Nash

HYOSCYAMUS NIGER: It is very useful in a form of dry cough which is aggravated when lying down and relieved by sitting up.

Dr. E. B. Nash

MEDORRHINUM: I have experimented more with the so-called nosodes and have had seemingly very good results from this remedy as well as Syphilinum in intractable cases of chronic rheumatism. The most characteristic difference between them is that with Medorrhinum the pains are worse in the day-time, and with Syphilinum in the night.

Dr. E. B. Nash

LYCOPODIUM: It will throw out a greater amount of eruption at first, but this will subside finally and the child will return to health.

Dr. J. T. Kent

In dropsy after the malaria Natrum mur., when it acts curatively, generally brings back the original chill.

Dr. J. T. Kent

All the Kalis are aggravated after any disturbance in fluid balance in the body, particularly after coition.

Dr. Donald A. Davis

In Psoriasis the first influence of Arsenicum is to make the eruption redder and more inflamed. This fact if not known, would lead to the suspension of the medicine just when it commenced to do good; at the same time, it is unnecessary to give it in doses sufficiently large to do this.

Dr. Ringer

When a patient is aggravated by Sulphur, we must always think of the existence of a latest state of syphilis, if Pulsatilla, another antidote of Sulphur does not produce any result.

Dr. Leon Renard

You can avoid aggravation from high potency by giving it three doses two hours apart.

Dr. T. K. Moore

SULPHUR: So strong is this affinity of Sulphur for the skin that it seems bent on pushing everything internal out on the surface.

Dr. E. B. Nash

SEPIA: This is to be given in the evening because if given in the morning, it may produce a sufficient aggravation to leave the patient feeling quite unless for that day.

Dr. R. A. F. Jack

After a prescription giving relief, do not give a remedy for any new symptoms appearing in a less vital part.

Dr. Adolph Lippe

It is prime rule not to keep repeating your remedy when the intervals between aggravations of the disease are lengthening. This is an indication that the patient is improving.

Homoeo Recorder, Aug. 31

VERATURM ALBUM: It is said to be a good remedy for rheumatism, which is worse in wet weather and which drives the patient out of bed.

Dr. E. B. Nash

ZINCUM MET.: A tedious aggravation in the convulsion and fever and a continuous brain cry is to be expected if a perfect cure is to result after administration of Zincum met.

Dr. J. T. Kent

9. CAUTIONS IN HOMOEOPATHY

ACONITUM NAPELLUS: The custom of alternating Aconite and Belladonna in inflammatory affections, which so widely prevails is a senseless one. Both remedies cannot be indicated at a time, and if a good effect follows their administration you may be sure that the indicated one cured in spite of the action of the other, which only hindered; or that the patient recovered without help from either.

Dr. E. B. Nash

ACONITUM NAPELLUS: So-called homoeopaths have fallen into similar error by concluding that because Aconite did quickly cure in some cases having a high grade of fever, that therefore it was always the remedy with which to treat cases having high fever. They even fell into the routine habit of prescribing this remedy for the first stage of all inflammatory affections, and follow it with other remedies more appropriate to the whole case further on.

Dr. E. B. Nash

ACONITUM NAPELLUS: Aconite is never to be given first to subdue the fever and then some other remedy 'to meet the case,' never to be alternated with other drugs for the purpose, as is often alleged, of 'controlling the fever.' If the fever be such as to require Aconite, no other drug is needed. If other drugs seem indicated, one should be sought which meets the fever as well, for many drugs besides Aconite produce fever, each after its kind."

Dr. Carrol Dunham

APIS 1M should be cautiously given during first three

months of pregnancy in low potencies, liable to produce miscarriage.

Dr. Comperthwaite

ARSENICUM ALBUM: Arsenicum is one of our best remedies for fevers of a typhoid character. So useful is it that Baehr says:—"Since Arsenic is, more than any other remedy, adapted to the worst forms of infectious diseases it seems wrong to delay its administration until the symptoms indicating it are developed in their most malignant intensity," and further, "Cur advice, therefore, is that Arsenic should be given more frequently than has been customary from the very beginning of the attack, and that we should not wait until the disease has fully developed its pernicious character." I do not think this is sound reasoning or good advice, for I have never found any rule by which I could decide from the beginning that a case would later on develop into a case of a pernicious or malignant character which would ever call for the exhibition of Arsenic. While we need not wait for a case to develop to that "most malignant" intensity which calls for Arsenic, we would not on the other hand be justified in giving Arsenic or any other remedy in anticipation of a condition which might never come. Arsenicum is not the only remedy capable of curing these malignant cases, and how do we know after all that it may not be Muriatic acid or Carbo vegetabilis that will be the remedy after the case is developed. There is no safe or scientific rule but to treat the case with the indicated remedy at any and all stages of the disease, without trying to treat expected conditions or future possibilities.

Dr. E. B. Nash

The general practitioner confronted with a case exhibiting

anaemia must avoid the temptation to commence treatment before making a diagnosis, for even single dose of a hae-matinic may entirely alter the marrow picture within twenty-four hours.

Dr. Charles Seward

BERBERIS: The remedy i.e. indicated for the patient will cure the patient, and the fistula. Above all things, they should not be operated on. To close up that fistulous opening, and thus neglect the patient, is a very dangerous thing to do. Knowing all that I now, if such a trouble should come upon me and I could not find the remedy to cure it I would bear with it patiently, knowing I was keeping a much less grievance. Nor could I advise my patient to have a thing done that I would not have done upon myself. It is a dangerous thing to operate upon fistula in another. It is a very serious matter. If it is closed up, and that patient is leaning towards phthisis, he will develop pathisis; if he has a tendency towards Bright's disease, that will hasten it; if he threatens to break down in any direction, his weakest parts will be affected, and he will break down. Occasionally time enough elapses so that the physician who is ignorant does not see the relation between the two. But now that you have heard it, you can never forget it.

Dr. J. T. Kent

BRYONIA: When patients are under constitutional reme-dies, they need caution about certain kinds of food that are known to disagree with their constitutional remedy. A Bryonia patient is often made sick from eating sauer krant, from vegetable salads, chicken salad, etc., so that you need not be surprised, after administering a dose of Bryonia for a constitutional state, to have your patient come in and say she has been made very ill from eating some one of these things. It is well to caution persons who are under the influence of Pulsatilla to avoid the use of fat foods, because very often they will upset the action of the remedy is similar to the patient when you administer it, and the things that he is to have are to be in agreement with that remedy.

Dr. J. T. Kent

'Coffee' must never be used when Chamomilla or Nux is the remedy. It would be equally true if you are treating a nervous paralytic with Causticum.

Dr. J. T. Kent

COCCUS CACTI: If he can lie in a cool room without much covering he will go longer without coughing.

Dr. J. T. Kent

CUPRUM MET: In that way a very poor prescriber may hunt around and get one remedy for one group of symptoms and other remedy for another group, and the patient be worse off than before. If the remedies are similar as to their general nature, then the little syperficial symptoms are not so extremely important.

Dr. J. T. Kent

EUPATORIUM PERF: The time for the administration of this dose is at the close of the paroxysm. You get the best effect when reaction is at the best, that is when reaction is setting in, after a paroxysm has passed off. That is true of every paroxysm disease, when it is possible to wait until the end.

Dr. J. T. Kent

It is better to know what you have done if you have killed your patient, than to be ignorant of it and go on and kill some more in the same way.

Dr. J. T. Kent

FLUORIC ACID: There are cases that would be greatly injured by so deeply acting a remedy as Silicea if given in the beginning, i.e, the suffering would be unnecessary; but if you commence with Pulsatilla you can mitigate the case and prepare it to receive Silicea, providing the two would appear to be on a plane of agreement. A very serious case had better first receive Pulsatilla, and the way being pared by that remedy follow it up with Silicea.

Dr. J. T. Kent

FERRUM METALLICUM: Iron is no more a panacea for anaemia than is Quinine for malaria or Phosphate of Lime for deficient bone development. My experience has taught me that there are several other equally efficient remedies for these conditions and that when they are not indicated they not only cannot cure but do injure every time they are prescribed, especially in the material doses in which they are generally recommended by such teachers. I must here state my experience founded on abundant practice and observation that such prescribing is not only un-Hahnemannian, but in every sense unhomoeopathic, and I warn all beginners not to practice along that line or they too will come to talk of the few satisfactory and certain things in modern medicine.

Dr. E. B. Nash

HEPAR SULPH: If our medicines were not powerful enough to kill folks, they would not be powerful enough to cure sick folks. It is well for you to realize that you are dealing with razors when dealing with high potencies. I would rather be in a room with a dozen negroes slashing with razors than in the hands of an ignorant prescriber of high potencies. They are means of tremendous harm, as well as of tremendous good.

Dr. J. T. Kent

HELLEBORUS NIGER: When it was given, repair set in; not instantly, but gradually. The remedy acts slowly in these slow, stubborn, stupid cases of brain and spinal trouble. Sometimes there is no apparent change until the day after the remedy is administered or even the next night, when there comes a sweat, a diarrhoea, or vomiting—a reaction. They must not be interfered with, no remedy must be given. They are signs of reaction. If the child has vitality enough to recover, he will now recover. If the vomiting is stopped by any remedy that will stop it, the Helleborus will be antidoted.

Dr. J. T. Kent

HEPAR SULPH: It is only very rarely that you will be able with your medicines to cure a stricture after it has taken on permanency, after it is many years old, but as long as the inflammation keeps up there is hope.

Dr. J. T. Kent

IODIUM: The local application for glandular enlargement is foolish and dangerous.

Dr. E. B. Nash

LACHESIS: It is recommended in epilepsy and locomotor

ataxia, but I have never seen good effects from it.

Dr. E. B. Nash

In old gouty cases, in old cases of Bright's disease, in advanced cases of pathisis where there are many tubercles, beware of Kali carb. given too high.

Dr. J. T. Kent

HYOSCYAMUS NIGER: It is also very useful in scarlatina of the typhoid form, and is complementary to Rhus tox. in those cases. I never alternate the two, but if the depressed sensorium and delirium goes beyond the power of Rhus to control I suspend the Rhus for a day or two and give Hyoscyamus, which will so improve the case that Rhus may again come into use and carry it to a successful termination. This is the only alternation I am ever guilty of. It is like that of Hahnemann when he alternated Bryonia and Rhus in fevers.

Dr. E. B. Nash

LAC DEFLORATUM: Many people are made sick by milk who use cream with safety and delight. Lac defloratum is often the remedy for such patients and after a careful examination their symptoms appear like the proving of skimmed milk.

Dr. J. T. Kent

IGNATIA: It is best to administer the dose in the morning if there is no occasion for hurry; when given shortly before bed time, it causes too much restlessness at night.

Dr. Samuel Hahnemann

The best time for taking an anti-psoric is in the morning before breakfast.

Dr. Samuel Hahnemann

In acute cases, one must have a remedy of the highest rating in the outstanding symptoms.

Dr. J. Stephenson

NUX VOMICA: Nux vomica will neither antidote the effects of the drug poison nor cure the disease condition unless it is homoeopathically indicated, especially if given in the dynamic form.

Dr. E. B. Nash

NUX VOMICA: No physician would be justified in prescribing Nux vomica on temperament alone, be the indication ever so clear. The whole case must come in.

Dr. E. B. Nash

Nux vomica acts best when given at night, during repose of mind and body; Sulphur in the morning.

Dr. E. B. Nash

OPIUM: There is no response to light, touch, noise or anything else, except the indicated remedy, which is Opium. So in pneumonia, where Opium has made remarkable cures in homoeopathic hand; while in massive, or what they like to all heroic, doses of the old school (given to stop pain and procure sleep) it has sent many a poor victim to his long resting place.

Dr. E. B. Nash

ARNICA: The sugar pills safely, permanently and gently, while the Quinine never curse, but suppresses, and there is nothing in the after history of that patient drugged with Quinine and Arsenic but congestion and voilence so long as he lives.

Dr. J. T. Kent

PHOSPHORUS: Beware of giving it in impotency or in weakness, as this is often associated with very feeble constitutions, and Phosphorus not only fails to cure, but seems to add to the weakness. Phosphorus will set patients to running down more rapidly who are suffering from vital weakness, who are always tired, simply weak, always prostrated and want to go to bed.

Dr. J. T. Kent

Psorinum patient does not improve while **coffee.**

Dr. P. Banerjee

Phosphorus, Silicea and Lachesis are three very dangerous remedies if there is pre-tubercular tendency. The wrong potency or too frequent repetition may drive the patient into an active tuberculosis.

Dr. E. W. Hubbard

The deeper remedies ought to be avoided if the vital force is low. Hahnemann warned against the use of Phosphorus in such cases of deficient vitality.

Dr. J. T. Kent

Always conserve the strength of your patient and never repeat a remedy which exhausts him.

Homoeo. Recorder, Aug. 31

After a prescription giving relief, do not give a remedy for any new symptoms appearing is a less vital part.

Dr. Adolph Lippe

Anti-psorics are apt to do harm in active syphilis, i.e. as long as the syphilis is the upper most miasm. But many anti-psorics are also anti-syphilitics, and they are not to be excluded as a rule.

Dr. J. T. Kent

The safe rule is, where there is definite improvement and continuous, nature has got the matter in hand, so just put yours behind you till the reappearance of symptoms demand further attention.

Dr. M. L. Tyler

In Enteric fever, when the temperature comes down to normal and even sub-normal, without any serious condition, don't give a remedy, since that will cause relapse.

Dr. Boger

Most of the symptoms in Causticum are aggravated from drinking coffee. You should therefore not allow patients to drink this beverage while taking Causticum.

Dr. Boger

When a nosode comes out in repertorizing, use it with care. it proves to be the similimum.

Dr. James Stephenson

It is well-known fact that any sort of prophylactic potentised or crude, falling within the incubation period of any infection often not only fails, but leads to virulent even fatal aggravation.

Dr. J. N. Kanjilal

The routine prescriber gives Belladonna to a child who has hot head, hot face and throbbing carotids and when it does not help he gives more Belladonna, and increases and size of his dose until the child has a proving.

Dr. J. T. Kent

Whenever treating a severe form of disease and an eruption comes to the surface, like a carbuncle or erysipelas, and does not give relief to the patient then there is danger. A remedy must be found soon.

Dr. J. T. Kent

All the symptoms should be examined between the attacks, so that the child may be elevated above these attacks because the acute remedy will do no more than suit the first, or second, or third at most.

Dr. J. T. Kent

There may be conditions in the human race that we, as yet, know no remedy for. We see certain groups of peculiar symptoms frequently repeat themselves and we know they are representatives of a state of the economy, but up to this day we may not have seen in the Materia Medica their counterpart. In medicines we have the exact counterpart for the diseases of the human race.

Dr. J. T. Kent

RHUS TOX: Rhus and Arsenicum are often indicated in typhoids, Aconite seldom or never, but all three are equally restless remedies.

Dr. E. B. Nash

RHUS TOX: Rhus is no less valuable in chronic skin troubles than in acute. Eczemas of the vesicular type are often cured by it; there is much itching which is not greatly relieved by scratching.

Dr. E. B. Nash

I stress the great danger of Aspirin and all Aspirin type drugs, even Alka-Seltzer, in people liable to peptic ulcer. Every year, we see at least one case and sometimes two or three with quite severe haematemesis from this cause, often requiring transfusion. The risk is especially great in febrile states, influenza etc., where gastritis is already present, and Aspirin sets up acute ulcerations not demonstrable on x-rays but capable of causing even fatal haemorrhage.

Dr. T. D. Rose

I am never very happy about leaving gall stones, specially if the gall-bladder is inflamed because of the danger of gall stone ileus. A stone ulcerating through into the duodenum may pass down the small intestine causing great damage and a most cheating type of intestinal intermittent obstruction often leading to gangrene of a large section of bowel.

Dr. T. D. Rose

KALI CARB: It would sometimes be cruel to give a dose of Kali carb. when the colic is on, because if the remedy fitted the case constitutionally, if all the symptoms of the case were those of Kali carb. you would be likely to get an aggravation that would be unnecessary. There are plenty of short acting remedies that would relieve the pain speedily, and at the close of the attack the constitutional remedy could then be given.

Dr. J. T. Kent

In advanced cases of Phthisis with early morning diarrhoea, when Sulphur is indicated but which aggravates if given, this medicine is useful: Rumex crisp.

Dr. J. T. Kent

If you are treating a case of syphilis with gumma in the brain where it is likely to be present in the later stage of syphilis, Ferrum might produce apoplexy, because of the already friable condition of the blood vessels. Then avoid Ferrum in tuberculosis, syphilis and in persons predisposed to haemorrhages and especially never repeat it.

Dr. J. T. Kent

KALI CARB: Do not be afraid to give the anti-psoric remedies when there is a history of tuberculosis in the family, but be careful when the patient is so far advanced with tuberculosis that there are cavities in the lung, or latent tubercles, or encyated caseous them, and some day after practicing while and making numerous mistakes in attempting to cure incurables you will admit the awful power of homoeopathic medicines.

Dr. J. T. Kent

Phosphorus will set patients to running down more rapidly who are suffering from a vital weakness, who was always fired, simple weak, always prostrated and want to go to bed.

Dr. J. T. Kent

PODOPHYLLUM: It is a common feature after giving a high potency of Podophyllum in a diarrhoea, that a headache comes on after the diarrhoea is stopped, It means that the medicine has acted suddenly and the headache will pass away soon.

Dr. J. T. Kent

RUTA: If the diarrhoea is very exhausting use some simple medicine, like this one, to slack it up. But the phthisical patient is better off with a little diarrhoea, a loose morning stool. It is the same with night sweat; if he does not have them he will have something more violent.

Dr. J. T. Kent

SECALE CORNUTUM: I fully agree with Cowerthwaite, who says: "To give it in parturition to hasten delivery, as is the practice of the old school, is simply inexcusable." On the other hand, I agree with Dr. H. N. Guernsey, "that it is useful when labor pains are weak, suppressed or distressing, in weak, cachectic women, in the 200th dilution," and have verified it beyond question.

Dr. E. B. Nash

SECALE CORNUTUM: Weak pains remedied by the indicated homoeopathic drug bring on natural labor, while large doses for the same purpose of an unindicated one do not and never can produce natural labor. It is nothing more or less than drug poisoning.

Dr. E. B. Nash

10. COMPLEMENTARY
AND
INIMICALS

ARSENICUM ALBUM: It often follows well after Mercurius, if that remedy only partially relieves.

Dr. E.B. Nash

ARGENTUM NITRICUM: Cuprum metallicum has great restlessness between the attacks. Finally, Natrum muriaticum is the best antidote for the abuse of Argentum nit., especially upon mucous surfaces.

Dr. E.B. Nash

COLCHICUM AUTUMNALE: It is always set down in the text-books for rheumatism, articular, migrating and gouty, and I have often tried it, but never with anything like the success of our other rheumatic remedies. I have been greatly disappointed in it here.

Dr. E.B. Nash

CARBO VEGETABILIS: Acidity and pyrosis is frequent; the plainest food disagrees, fat foods especially. Here Carbo vegetabilis succeeds when Pulsatilla fails.

Dr. E.B. Nash

China and **Carbo vegetabilis** are decidedly complementary.

Dr. E.B. Nash

Coffea does not relieve, follow with Chamomilla.

Dr. E.B. Nash

COFFEA CRUDA: Hering used to recommend Aconite and

Coffea in alternation in painful inflammatory affections where the fever symptoms of the former and also the nervous sensibility of the latter were present, and I know of no two remedies that alternate better, though I never do it, since I learned to closely individualize.

Dr. E.B. Nash

Cadmium Sulph: and **Phosphorus** are antidotes to Radium burns in case of treatment of carcinoma by radiation. Give 1M.

Dr. R.B. Das

Colocynthis cures colics again and again. Then Kali carb steps to end the troubles.

Dr. T.K. Moore

CARBO VEGETABILIS: China is its great complementary

Dr. E.B. Nash

CALCAREA OSTREARUM: Very many cases in the incipient stage come within range of Sulphur or Calcarea.

Dr. E.B. Nash

HAMAMELIS VIRGINICA: I am not in favour, generally of using remedies in this way, unless it be for external injuries, which are not diseases.

Dr. E.B. Nash

FERRUM METALLICUM: It is evident, therefore, that iron does not act as a curative agent by virtue of its absorption as a constituent of the blood, but rather, as we are led conclude, from its physiological effects upon the organs and tissues of the body, that it owes its therapeutic virtues to the same essential dynamic agency possessed by other drugs, and its application is subject to the same therapeutic law.

Dr. E.B. Nash

IGNATIA: Ignatia bears the same relation to the diseases of women that Nux does to bilious men.

Dr. E.B. Nash

KALI HYDROIODICUM: Hepar sulphur. is one of the best antidotes. Most of the reported cures with this remedy Kali iod. are made with the low or crude preparations of the durg.

Dr. E.B. Nash

KALI HYDROIODICUM: When the remedy is not similar enough to cure in such a form the increasing of the dose does not make it homoeopathic. There is an idea in vogue that increasing the dose makes the remedy similar. That is going away from principle. If the remedy is not similar there is no form of dose that can make it similar.

Dr. J.T. Kent

If Lycopodium symptomatically prescribed gives no results, give Luesinum, which is its best complementary.

Dr. Fergiewoods

NATRUM SULPHURICUM: Sulphur drives the patient out of bed, but Natrum sulph., like Bryonia, is worse only after beginning to move.

Dr. E.B. Nash

In my experience, Psorinum is often indicated after Pyrogen.

Dr. E. Underhill

Siliceas is the chronic of Pulsatilla.

Dr. E.B. Nash

SEPIA: I should give Causticum after Phosphorus, Silicea after Mercury, or Rhus tox. after Apis mel. if I found them indicated.

Dr. E.B. Nash

SULPHUR: I think Arsenicum leads in all acute diseases, while Sulphur leads in chronic affections.

Dr. E.B. Nash

SULPHUR: Bryonia and Sulphur complement each other; but, of course, the symptoms must decide and may decide in favour of neither of them.

Dr. E.B. Nash

11. DIOGNOSIS THROUGH SYMPTOMS

Any child with an un-explained pallor, pyrexia, malaise or ill health of several weeks or months duration, should be suspected of having tubercular infection.

Dr. Balgopal Raju

The more experience I have with the use of cadmium preparations the more convinced I am of their indispensable need in Cancer.

Dr. A.H. Grimmer

Suppurative condition about the root of the nails suggest the digestive upset whether it is a gall bladder or liver upset or whether it is an Appendix—the patients are liable with the attack concurrently.

Dr. D.M. Borland

Dreaming of flying is an indication of vaccinal poisoning.

Dr. Ellis Barker

In cases without symptoms, the patient must be kept on sac lac until you can discern some general such as aggravation of symptoms in the evening or at midnight.

If the patient is only 'tired' without guiding symptoms, you may know that it is liable to termination in some grave disorder, tuberculosis, Bright's disease, cancer or the like.

Dr. V.R. Carr

The triad of severe headache, fever and vomiting should at once raise the suspicion of Meningitis, for, in no disease is early diagnosis more important.

Dr. Charles Seward

Carcinoma of the rectum is a common disease and must be suspected in all patients who have persistent rectal bleeding; proctitis or procto-colitis should always be suspected when there is persistent rectal bleeding in young people.

Dr. Parke

Causticum: Dryness of the mouth and throat; rawness of the throat; must swallow constantly nervous feeling in throat. This is often a fore-runner of paralysis.

Dr. J.T. Kent

Oedema in the absence of dyspnoea or cardiac enlargement, is not due to heart disease.

Dr. S. Sen

When children are sick and show no clearly defined cause for illness, the ears should be invariably examined for probable infection.

Dr. H.S. Weaver

In epilepsy, the remedy is not seen in the actual seizure (pathological symptom) but rather in what has preceded perhaps long before.

Dr. R.O. Spalding

A history of recurring lumbago, sciatica or fibrositis, especially in young men with stiffness of back; poor chest movement and perhaps iritis should call spondylitis in mind.

Dr. Charles Seward

No head injury is so slight that it should be neglected, or so evere that life should be despaired of.

Dr. Bailey & Dr. Bishop

Abrupt loss of consciousness without faintness, sweating or palpitation, even if not preceded by any sensory aura, is almost certainly epileptic.

Dr. C. Kennedy

Lower abdominal pain, backache, and rheumatism in distant parts of the body in women, have been attributed to a cervical infection and the **cervix** has been described as the **pelvic tonsil.**

Dr. Bryan Williams

The dictum 'no acid, no ulcer' holds good in nearly all cases of peptic ulcer, and an ulcer, without free acid, suggests the presence of Carcinoma.

Dr. Ivy

With rare exceptions, patients with heart disease rarely faint.

Dr. S. Sen

Any irregular bleeding from the uterus is abnormal and must indicate a presumptive diagnosis of Carcinoma; this is particularly so at the climacteric.

Dr. Tomkinson

At all ages, any abdominal pain that has continued without intermission for several hours must be regarded as possible Appendicitis, especially if it is associated with vomiting.

Dr. John Fry

Unexplained numbness of the chin and lower lip must be considered an ominous indication of grave disease. (Carcinoma).

Dr. J.R. Calverley

Coldness of one foot suddenly occurring after an operation may be sign of a "silent heart attack."

Dr. Nathan Frank

A large liver, jaundice and a normal spleen point to gall stones or cancer; but if the spleen is also enlarged, it suggests cirrhosis of liver or portal obstruction. A very enlarged spleen with but slightly enlarged liver suggests some of the blood diseases and needs blood examination.

Dr. S.Sen

Tuberculosis women of the Phosphorus type readily abort.

Dr. Ellis Barker

To avoid backache; one rule of thumb: A woman should never lift more than 25 lbs, and a man should never lift more than half his weight.

Today's Health

Any obstinate catarrh that resist Tuberculinum b. and other remedies, should be investigated for intestinal toxaemia (for using bowel nosodes).

Dr. C.R. Wheeler

Sycotic children (so born) when one or both patients have

Gonorrhoea, have Cholera infantum, marasmus pining children.

Dr. J.T. Kent

Always be suspicious of a sudden cessation of symptoms without a reaction. If the patient gets better almost instantly with no sign of a reaction, if arouses the suspicion that the action of the remedy is only palliative.

Dr. Boger

It kills the Psoric patients to stand still; he must walk even if he is on his feet but for a brief time; weakness of the ankle joints is a sure indication of the presence of combined Syphilitic and Psoric miasms.

Dr. H.A. Roberts

The Psoric patient is always conscious of his heart condition and it is he who takes his own pulse.

Dr. H.A. Roberts

Psora alone produces more marked anasarcas and dropsies than Syconsis; the sycotic patient succumbs before the dropsical condition becomes marked; but the union of the two miasms produced these conditions in a marked degrees.

Dr. H.A. Roberts

In Rheumatoid Arthritis : the fingers and hands are stiff on soking in the morning and the stiffness is relieved by soking them in hot water.

In the Arthritis sometimes met with in Myxoedema, which may be mistaken for Rheumatoid Arthritis, there is no early morning stiffness, the patient complaining of swelling, numbness and tingling.

Dr. Beaumont

Tuberculosis of the spine is the most important cause of spigastric pain of extra-abdominal origin. It must specially be remembered in children.

Dr. Charles Seward

The persistence of intense jaundice in an old man for over 5 to 7 weeks without any other cause should be suspected as cancer.

Dr. S. Sen

Subnormal temperature, pulse and respiration with stupor occurring in the course of a middle ear discharge indicates brain abscess.

Dr. George W. Mackenzie

In extravasation of urine, a black patch on the penis is a harbinger of death.

Dr. B. Bordie

The appearance of albumin and disappearance of sugar in the urine, of a diabetic is an ominous sign and suggests a grave prognosis. It is an evidence of severe kidney's damage due to the constant excertion of sugar.

Dr. Chari

Any previously healthy child, especially between two months and two years of age, who is suddenly seized with sharp intermittent abdominal pain and vomiting, should be regarded as suffering from intersusception and sent to hospital without delay.

Dr. Donald Court

It is very rare to find a clean tongue in a case of acute obstructive appendicitis.

Dr. Milnes Walker

In all cases of retracted nipple in young women, suspect latent ovarian disease.

Homoeopathic Recorder

Excessive crying in babies: A clinical examination is always necessary and particular attention should be paid to the ears, and the urine, since otitis media and pyelitis often occur silently in babies.

Dr. Cohn Fry

A very common observation which has been made is that obese patients practically never develop diabetic coma whilst a thin emaciated juvenile diabetic easily develop diabetic coma.

Dr. Chari

Diabetes and tuberculosis are frequently found to exist together. Tuberculosis is far advanced when detected in diabetic patients.

Dr. Helden

Some put their arms up above the head while sleeping. When

they sleep like that, they always have liver disease; always have congestion of liver. There is some trouble with liver. But in children it is normal. In adults, it is not so.

Dr. Piere Schmidt

With an extensive coronary thrombosis, the blood pressure may be so low that no urine is secreted—this is a very serious symptom.

Dr. Beaumont

KALI HYDROIODICUM: The frothy expectoration is found in oedema of the lungs and may occur in Bright's disease.

Dr. E.B. Nash

KALI HYDROIODICUM: Remember that both subjective and objective symptoms must enter into every case in order to make the totality complete.

Dr. E.B. Nash

LILIUM TIGRINUM: The uterine symptoms are sometimes marked so as to be over-looked for the time by the violence of the heart symptoms.

Dr. E.B. Nash

STANNUM: A certain physician in Albany, N.Y., was called in consultation on a so-called case of phthisis pulmonalis. The case was in allopathic hands. After carefully examining the case, he was asked: "What is your diagnosis, doctor?" "Stannum," said the doctor. "What! :" "Stannum," replied the doctor. Stannum was the diagnosis of the remedy, not the disease. It was given and cured the patient.

Dr. E.B. Nash

PHOSPHORIC ACID: It seems very singular that, after so much talk about the general depression or weakness of this remedy, we should be obliged to record that the profuse and sometimes long-continued diarrhoea should not debilitate, as a characteristic symptoms.

Dr. E.B. Nash

12. SOME RENEDIES OF SPECIFIC NATURE

ANTIMONIUM TARTARICUM: The nausea of this remedy is as intense as that of Ipecacuanha, but not so persistent, and there is relief after vomiting. I have found it nearest a specific (of course we know there is no absolute specific for any disease) for cholera morbus of any remedy. For more than 25 years, I have seldom found it necessary to use any other, and then only when there were severe cramps in the stomach and bowels, when Cuprum metallicum relieved.

Dr. E.B. Nash

AURUM METALLICUM: Aurum is one of the few remedies that has hemiopia or half-sight, and has cured it even in the 200th potency. Lycopodium and Lithium carbonicum also have half-sight, but Aurum sees only the lower, while the other two see only the left half of objects.

Dr. E.B. Nash

ACONITUM NAPELLUS: It has two very important modalities, viz., fright and dry cold air.

Dr. E.B. Nash

AURUM METALLICUM: I once cured a young lady who tried to commit suicide by drowning. After she was cured she laughed at the occurrence, and said she could not help it. It seemed to her she was of no use in the world. She left so

Dr. E.B. Nash

AURUM METALLICUM: You take away a man's hope and he has nothing to live for, he then wants to die. Such it seems, is the state in this medicine.

Dr. J.T. Kent

ARSENICUM ALBUM: I once had a case of very severe gastralgia caused by suppression of eczema on the hands. I knew nothing of the suppression, but prescribed Arsenicum because the pains came on at midnight, lasting until 3 A.M., during which time the patient had to walk the floor in agony, and there was great burning in the stomach. She had but one slight attack after taking Arsenicum, but, said she, when I visited her, "Doctor, would that remedy send out salt rheum?" Then I found out about the suppression which had been caused by the application of an ointment, and told her that she could have back the pain in the stomach any time she wanted it, by suppressing the eruption again. She did not want it.

Dr. E.B. Nash

ARSENICUM ALBUM: It is particularly efficacious in many affections of the lungs, where the breathing is very much oppressed. Respiration is wheezing, with cough and frothy expectoration. Patient cannot lie down; must sit up to breathe, and is unable to move without being greatly put out of breath. The air passages seem constricted. It is especially useful in asthmatic affections caused or aggravated by suppressed eruptions, like pneumonia from retrocedent measles, or even chronic lung troubles from suppressed eczema.

Dr. E.B. Nash

ASAFOETIDA: Asthmatic attacks at least once a day all her life, brought on by every bodily exertion, coition, especially by every satisfying meal.

Dr. J.T. Kent

ARGENTUM NITRICUM: Dyspepsia, gastralgia and even gastric ulcer have sometimes found a powerful remedy in Argentum, and it has also done great good in very obstinate cases of diarrhoea of various kinds.

Dr. E.B. Nash

ARNICA MONTANA: I have often relieved sewing girls or students of pains in the eyes from this cause and have sometimes enabled them to lay off the glasses that had been prescribed by the opticians. It is much better to use this remedy in a weakened power of accommodation than to try and compensate for it with artificial lenses. Or course where the impaired vision is purely optical this cannot be done.

Dr. E.B. Nash

ACTAEA RACEMOSA: Each women is a law into herself. In this remedy the sufferings are during menstrual flow as a rule.

Dr. J.T. Kent

AETHUSA: It is at the lead of the least of medicines for that conditions; that is, when digestion has absolutely ceased from brain trouble.

Dr. J.T. Kent

ALUMINA: She will continue to strain, covered with copious sweat, hanging on to the seat, if there be any place to hang on to, and will pull and work as if in labour, and at last is able to expel a soft stool, yet with the sensation that more stool remains.

Dr. J.T. Kent

ANTIMONIUM CRUDUM: It produces a very serious state in the mind, an absence of the desire to live.

Dr. J.T. Kent

ANTIMONIUM TARTARICUM: Dropsy is one of the natural conditions of all forms of Antimonium.

Dr. J.T. Kent

ARGENTUM MET: It has been an astonishing feature in this remedy that precisely at the hour of noon a great many troubles come on, and the pains and aches. Chills, headaches.

Dr. J.T. Kent

ARGENTUM MET: It cures albuminuria; it cures diabetes, with sugar in the urine; and many of the broken down conditions of the kidneys.

Dr. J.T. Kent

ARGENTUM MET: It is a medicine of great use in horribly offensive leucorrhoea. (Kali Ars., Kali Phos.)

Dr. J.T. Kent

ARSENICUM ALBUM: Arsenic and Merc-corr. are the two principal medicines for spreading ulcerations, such as eat in every direction, very offensive.

Dr. J.T. Kent

ASAFOETIDA: I never like to see them come into my

7

office, for they are hard cases to manage.

Dr. J.T. Kent

ARGENTUM MET: Where it was given in case of scirrhus of the uterus it says, "In less than three days foul smell was lost entirely." When a remedy acts in that manner it actually stops the growth. In fact, a cancerous state that would go on to its termination in 14 to 16 months will go two or three years and the patient remaims comfortable. The remedy i.e. indicated stops the ulceration, it checks the destruction, and keeps the patient comfort and with her friends for years.

Dr. J.T. Kent

AURUM METALLICUM: You take away a man's hope and he has nothing to live for, he then wants to die. Such, it seems, is the state in this medicine.

Dr. J.T. Kent

BELLADONNA has not the gradual rise and the gradual fall like a continued fever.

Dr. J.T. Kent

BELLADONNA is full of thirst, we find when we come to study the stomach symptoms.

Dr. J.T. Kent

BRYONIA: Every medicine has a sphere of action, a peculiar nature whereby it differs from all other medicines and hence it becomes suitable to complaints of one class and not suitable to those of another. It is like the nature of human beings, as they differ from each to her, and also like the nature of diseases, which differ from each other in character.

Dr. J.T. Kent

BUFO: We do have plenty of remedies for people who have epilepsy. A large percentage of the cases are curable.

Dr. J.T. Kent

BELLADONNA is the best remedy for stiff neck of rheumatic origin or from cold.

Dr. E. A. Farrington

BELLADONNA: It is astonishing how many local inflammations, even a carbuncle or boil, will so disturb the general system and circulation, as to produce the general inflammatory fever, with the characteristic head symptoms calling for Belladonna, and no less astonishing how this remedy controls the whole condition, both local and general, when indicated. What! exclaims the believer in local applications, give Belladonna internally for a boil on the hand or foot? Yes, indeed, not only Belladonna, but Mercurius, Hepar sulphuris, Tarentula cubensis, and many others, and you will not have any need for local medication at all.

Dr. E.B. Nash

CHAMOMILLA: There is a remedy for inflammation of the tonsils where the ear is envolved and is ameliorated by heat, that very few use, but it is of great value; it is Chamomilla, and it is especially indicated if the patient is irritable.

Dr. J.T. Kent

CALCAREA CARB: An opacity itself, when it is present,

is not a symptom, but a result of disease.

Dr. J.T. Kent

CALCAREA CARB: The Calcarea patient can't go upstairs; he is so tired in his legs, and so tired in the chest; he pants and suffocates from going upstairs. He has every evidence of muscular weakness and flabbiness. Nutrition is impaired everywhere. This is the kind of patient that used to be called scrofulous; now we call the condition psora; and Calcarea is one of our deepest anti-psoric. It is a medicine that goes deep into the life, and takes a deep hold of every part of the economy.

Dr. J.T. Kent

CALCAREA CARB: Any amount of thinking becomes impossible. It is almost impossible for him to come to a conclusion, for he never figures it twice alike.

Dr. J.T. Kent

CALCAREA CARB: When an individual ceases to love his own life, and is weary of it, and loathes it, and wants to die, he is on the border line of insanity. In fact, that is an insanity of the will you have only to look with an observing eye to see that one may be insane in the affections, or insane in the intelligence. One may remain quite intact, and the other one be destroyed.

Dr. J.T. Kent

CALCAREA CARB: The hair fall out, not in the regular way such as occurs in old age, but in patches here and there.

Dr. J.T. Kent

CALCAREA CARB: It is a peculiar feature of Calcarea, that the more marked the congestion of internal parts, the colder the surface becomes. With chest troubles, and stomach troubles, and bowel troubles, the feet and hands become like ice, and covered with sweat; and he lies in bed sometimes with a fever in the rest of his body, and the scalp covered with cold sweat.

Dr. J.T. Kent

CUPRUM tones down, relieves that sensitivity, and well selected remedies will then act curatively and long.

Dr. J.T. Kent

CARBO VEGETABILIS: No truer remark was ever written than that Carbo vegetabilis is especially adapted to cachectic individuals whose vital powers have become weakened. This remark is made particularly clear when considered in the light of those cases in which diseases seems to be engrafted upon the system by reason of the depressing influence of some prior derangement (Psorinum).

Dr. Henry N. Guernsey

CARBO VEGETABILIS: Of course, no remedy can raise the dead, no matter how strong the indications before death; but no remedy can come nearer than this and the dominant school know little or nothing about it, and never can until they will consent to use it in the homoeopathic form and according to homoeopathic indications.

Dr. E.B. Nash

CALCAREA OSTREARUM: We must not omit to notice the action of Calcarea ost. on the respiratory organs, for the reason that it is of great importance in its use in that dread disease, pulmonary consumption.

Dr. E.B. Nash

CALCAREA OSTREARM: It is one of the most effective agents, if indicated by the temperament and symptoms, in the cure of this malady, and if applied at a stage when a cure is at all possible.

Dr. E.B. Nash

CAULOPHYLLUM: I have given this remedy in long-continued passive haemorrhage from the uterus after miscarriage when I had the characteristic weakness and sense of internal trembling present.

Dr. E.B. Nash

CICUTA VIROSA: It is also a good remedy for the effects of concussion of the brain or spine, if spasms are in the train of chronic effects therefrom and Arnica does not relieve.

Dr. E.B. Nash

Whenever a medicine makes a man desire to do something it affects his will, and when it affects his intelligence it is acting on his understanding. Medicines act on both.

Dr. J.T. Kent

HYOSCYAMUS NIGER: If acute delirium passes on into the settled form, called mania, this remedy is still one of our chief reliances.

Dr. E.B. Nash

HYOSCYAMUS NIGER: "Every muscle in the body twitches, from the eyes to the toes." This is one of his chief indications for its use in convulsions, whether epileptic or not.

Dr. E.B. Nash

HELONIAS DIOICA: There is almost always associated with it a more or less anaemic condition. This anaemia may seem to be consequent upon too profuse menstruation or flooding, or it may exist entirely independent of any such cause. In these cases I have often found albumen present in the urine, sometimes in large quantities, especially in pregnant women, and seen rapid improvement and disappearance of the albumen under the action of this remedy.

Dr. E.B. Nash

IPECACUANHA: It is true that when patients have bled until they have become anaemic, and are subject to dropsy, Ipecacuanha to be the remedy; its natural follower then is China, which will bring the patient in a position to need an antipsoric remedy.

Dr. J.T. Kent

LACHESIS: In short, the circulation in Lachesis subjects is very uncertain. This is what makes it so valuable in sudden flushes during the climacteric period.

Dr. E.B. Nash

LYCOPODIUM: A feeling of satiety is found under this remedy which alternates with a feeling of hunger of a peculiar kind.

Dr. E.B. Nash

KALI HYDROIODICUM: 'Kali Iod' in the words of E.A. Farrington: "Pneumonia, in which disease it is an excellent remedy when hepatization has commenced, when the disease localizes itself, and infiltration begins. In such cases, in the absence of other symptoms calling distinctively for Bryonia, Phosphorus or Sulphur, I would advise you to select Iodine or Iodide of Potass. It is also called for when the hepatization is so extensive that we have cerebral congestion, or even an effusion into the brain as a result of this congestion.

Dr. E.B. Nash

DIGITALIS PURPUREA: A young man of good habits was taken with nausea and vomiting. He was drowsy, and after a couple of days he began to grow very jaundiced all over. The sclerotica were as yellow as gold, as was, indeed, the skin all over the body, even to the nails. The stools were natural as to consistence, but perfectly colourless, while the urine was as brown as lager beer, or even more so. Where you could see through it, on the edge of the receptacle, it was yellow as fresh bile. The pulse was only thirty beats per minute, and often dropped out a beat.

This was a perfect Digitalis cash of jaundice, and this remedy cured him perfectly in a few days, improvement in his feelings taking place very shortly after beginning it; the stools, urine and skin gradually taking on their natural colour. The characteristic slow, pulse was the leading symptoms to the prescription, for all the rest of the symptoms may be found in almost any well-developed case of severe jaundice.

Dr. E.B. Nash

NATRUM MURIATICUM: It is one of our best remedies for anaemia. It does not seem to make much difference whether the anaemia is caused by loss of fluids (China, Kali carb.), menstrual irregularities (Puls), loss of semen (Phos. acid, China), grief or other mental diseases.

Dr. E.B. Nash

NATRUM MURIATICUM: It is apt to occur after the menstrual period, as if caused by loss of blood, and you know that China also has throbbing headache in such cases. With Natrum the throbbing headache occurs whether the menses be scanty or profuse.

Dr. E.B. Nash

Opium & Glonoine: They equalize the circulation, and the patient may not die.

Dr. J.T. Kent

PODOPHYLLUM: I once made a brilliant cure of an obstinate case of intrermittent fever with this remedy. The chills were very violent and were followed by intense fever with great loquacity. There was also great jaundice present.

Dr. E.B. Nash

If you had a child with copious, gushing, violently foetid stool, ameliorated by lying on the abdomen, and it would have another stool if lying any other way, Podophyllum would be the remedy.

Dr. J.T. Kent

SULPHUR: Let no one understand that Sulphur is the only remedy capable of removing psoric complications, but simply that Sulphur will be likely to be oftener indicated here, because it oftener covers the usual manifestations of psora in its pathogenesis than any other remedy. There are anti-psorics, like Psorinum, Causticum, Graphites, etc., which may have to be used instead of Sulphur. And we know which one by the same law which guides us in the selection of the right remedy and time.

Dr. E.B. Nash

SULPHUR: No one need tell me that there is no relation of skin to internal troubles. I have seen too much of it, and have cured many cases of that character, where a restoration of the skin disease relieved the internal which had followed its retrocession or suppression.

Dr. E.B. Nash

SILICEA: It does not increase in size or strength, learns to walk late; in short, if not actually sick in bed, everything seems to have come to a standstill so far as growth or development is concerned.

Dr. E.B. Nash

SILICEA: It is the remedy to restore and cure such sweats by correcting the conditions upon which the sweats depend.

Dr. E.B. Nash

SECALE CORNUTUM: I have never, in a practice of 35 years, used it in this way, but have always been able to control such haemorrhages. Secale is not often indicated in active post-partum haemorrhages.

Dr. E.B. Nash

SPONGIA TOSTA: The dry, chronic, sympathetic cough of organic heart disease is oftener and more permanently relieved by this remedy than by Naja. Spongia is also a good remedy for goitre, with sense of suffocation after sleep.

Dr. E.B. Nash

SABADILLA: A sleepiness comes on from thinking, meditating, reading. While meditating in a chair he falls asleep like Nux moschata and phosphoric acid.

Dr. J.T. Kent

13. POTENCIES

ANTIMONIUM TARTARICUM: If Sulphur should not promote absorption in such a case, Tartar emetic will often do it. I have used it from the 200th to the cm. potencies with equally good results.

Dr. E.B. Nash

AURUM MET: Aurum is one of the few remedies that has hemiopia or half-sight, and has cured it even in the 200th potency.

Dr. E.B. Nash

ARGENTUM NITRICUM: Allen & Norton write as follows: "The greatest service that Argentum nitricum performs is in purulent ophthalmia. With large experience, in both hospital and private practice, we have not lost a single eye from this disease, and every one has been treated with internal remedies, most of them with Argentum nitricum of a high potency, 30th or 200th.

Dr. E.B. Nash

In addition to Antimonium crudum for corns in general, recent or painful corns, Ferrum pic. 3 is useful and very effective and for the constitutional tendency, Redium brom. 30 once a fortnight will give the patient a now lease of life.

Dr. Pettitt.

Never change a remedy that has done good, until you have given it in a higher potency.

Dr. Hughes

In high temperatures use the medium potency 200th and repeat night and morning until reaction occurs.

Dr. Boger

BAPTISIA TINCTORIA: I have used both the low and high preparations with equal success, but now use the 30th potency.

Dr. E.B. Nash

For hyper sensitive patients, use low or medium potencies.

Dr. Stuart Clouse

High potencies will not palliate incurable cases; you must use the low.

Dr. Boger

Some 80% or fever blisters can be quickly cured often in 36 hours with Natrum mur. in 6x, 12x or 30th potencies. I have seen some cases of fever blisters cured as if magic with Rananculus bulb., or Rananculus-s., which would not respond to Natrum mur. in any potency.

Dr. E. Petrie Hoyle

Ganglions were dispersed by Benzoic acid given internally in the dilutions from the 12th and the 30th.

Dr. Turrel

We have repeatedly proved its value in fevers apparently simple, but which failed to yield to Aconite. It should be given in a low dilution the 1x or even the strong tincture.

Dr. Ruddock

I use Bacillinum 30 in incipient tuberculosis. In early cases, it is my custom to give a dose once every 10 days to two weeks. I have had many early cases that cleared up after a few months treatment with this preparation. In late stage of tuberculosis, Bacillinum is of no benefit.

Dr. Walter Sands Mills

When reaction is delayed in distressing crisis after a potency as low as the 200th or 1M has been given, go to the 50M or higher and grateful relief will ensue.

Dr. R.E.S. Hayes

In acute conditions, never give more than three doses of a remedy in the same potency. If patient is much better or worse after any one dose do not repeat. Later it may be necessary to repeat the remedy in a higher potency.

Homoeo. Recorder, June 28

You do not build mole hills out of our high potencies; they simply establish a state of order, so that digestion and assimilation go on, order is established and the tissues are improved. Health comes, beauty, a growth of hair, better skin, better nails.

Dr. J.T. Kent

CANNABIS SATIVA: I used them all in the cm., and I know, having tried both, that they cure better than the low potencies.

Dr. E.B. Nash

CINCHONA OFFICINALIS: China will do excellent service. It is equally good in splenic diseases which closely resemble the splenic troubles resulting from the abuse of Quinine. I have found the 200th do better than lower

COFFEA CRUDA: Coffea has won to itself great credit as a sleep remedy. In my experience and observation, it works best here in the 200th potency.

CAULOPHYLLUM: I concluded to try Caulophyllum high. I did so in the 200th potency and cured the whole case promptly and permanently.

CICUTA VIROSA: I once had a case of eczema capitis in a young woman-it was of long standing-which covered the whole scalp, solid, like a cap. I gave her Cicuta 200th and cured her completely in a very short time.

CAMPHOR: Camphor is the first remedy to be thought of, and according to susceptibility or strength of the patient the dose must be varied from tincture to highest potency.

MERCURIUS SOLUBILIS: I used in my early practice to put five drops mother tincture into four ounces of water (in a four ounce vial) and let the patient take a teaspoonful three times a day. After about four days the inflammatory symptoms would have subsided, and the thin discharge have thickened and become greenish in appearance. Then Mercurius solubilis 3d trituration, a powder three times a day, would often finish the case. Or if a little, thin, gleety discharge remained, I cured that with Sulphur, Capsicum or Kali iodide. I have cured many cases in from one to two weeks this way. Later I have used the c.m. potency in the first stage, and sometimes never have to use the second remedy.

Dr. E.B. Nash

GELSEMIUM NITIDUM: I consider the large doses of either remedy used by some to quiet excited conditions, or to control spasms or convulsions by their toxic, depressing, or paralyzing action on the muscular system, antipathic, and in no way truly curative. I have never known the remedy to do much good in these conditions below the 30th potency, but often in the potencies much above that.

Dr. E.B. Nash

In varicose veins of the leg, you will be delighted with the way in which the first or second dilution of Hamamelis will cure the pain.

Dr. Hughes

IGNATIA: In one case of puerperal convulsions, other remedies having failed to do any good, the consulting physician while observing the patient during one of the spasms noticed that she came out of it with a succession of long drawn sighs. He inquired if the patient had any recent mental trouble, and learned that she had lost her mother, of whom she was exceedingly fond, and whom she had mourned for greatly, a few weeks before. Ignatia 30th quickly cured her.

Dr. E.B. Nash

IRIS VERSICOLOR: I used to give the remedy in the 3d; but of late years have given it in the 50m. and am better pleased with the result, because it is more prompt and lasting.

Dr. E.B. Nash

IPECACUANHA: It is a better remedy than Secale ever was or can be, for post-partum haemorrhages, and it is not necessary to use it in large and poisonous doses, for it will stop them in the 200th potency, and is quicker in its action than Secale.

Dr. E.B. Nash

IODIUM: I have cured many cases of goitre with Iodine c.m., when indicated, giving a powder every night for four nights, after the moon fulled and was waning.

Dr. E.B. Nash

KALI BICHROMICUM: I have with it cured many cases of diphtheritic croup, and of late years never give it below the 30th potency, because abundant experience has convinced me that it does better than the low triturations.

Dr. E.B. Nash

KALI HYDROIODICUM: I think it can be used lower than most drugs without injury, and yet I believe we do not know half its remedial power as developed by our process of potentisation.

Dr. E.B. Nash

KREOSOTUM: I have used it here also in the 200th. Kreosote is also one of our best remedies in other kinds of vomiting; in the vomiting of pregnancy and in that other intractable disease of the stomach, known as gastromalacia

Dr. E.B. Nash

One has seen Kreosote 200 annihilative of the terrible odours that sometimes accompany cancer of the cervix, where if it did nothing more, it made life more supportable for patient and for entourage.

Dr. M.L. Tyler

Gelsemium should never be forgotten in inveterate backache. It is recommended in doses all the way from 10 drops of Q to 10M.

Medical Century, 1893

KALI CARBONICUM: If you give Kali-carb, to one of the incurable patients in very high potency it will make your patient worse, and the aggravation will be serious and prolonged, but the 30th may be of great service.

Dr. J.T. Kent

KALI HYDROIODICUM: I used to dissolve two to four grains of the crude salt in a four ounce vial of water and direct to take a teaspoonful of this preparation three times a day, until it is half used, and then fill up with water and continue taking the same way until cured; filling up the vial every time of this description and feeling sure of my remedy, I gave it in the 200th potency as an experiment. This case also made fully as speedy a recovery as the others treated with the crude drug, so since then I often prescribe it in the potencies.

Dr. E.B. Nash

It is well for you to realise that you are dealing with razors when dealing with high potencies. I would rather be in the room with a dozen negroes slashing with razors than in the hands of an ignorant prescriber of high potencies. They are means of tremendous harm as well as of tremendous good.

Dr. J.T. Kent

STRAMONIUM: I cured a case just as bad since then with the cm. potency.

Dr. E.B. Nash

LAC CANINUM: Lac caninum cured the case very quickly. Not long after I had a very severe case of scarlatina.

The throat was swollen full, and restlessness was so marked with pains in the limbs which left the patient tossing from side to side that I thought surely Rhus tox. must be the remedy. But it failed to relieve. Then I discovered that the soreness of the throat and the pains alternated sides. This called my mind to the remedy, which was given with prompt relief. I used the cm. in this case.

Dr. E.B. Nash

SYPHILINUM: It is a cure of caries of the spine of long standing by Syphilinum (high). I had a very similar case, for which I had been prescribing for over a year without success, when I first read the report of this case. In my case, as in his, the patient had severe pains in the diseased part during the night. Every one acquinted with syphilitic troubles, especially of the bones, knows of these (terrible, sometimes) nightly bone pains. Three doses of Swan's Syphilinum cm. cured this case in the remarkably short space of 40 days.

Dr. E.B. Nash

One may prescribe on a pathological basis where a remedy

is known to have a relationship with certain tissues, for e.g. Hepar sulph. for suppuration, Silicea for inflammation near bone, Bryonia for serous tissues. The potency in pathological prescribing is important, for if the patient's vitality is low, a high potency may make too big demands on the system and harm rather than good come of it.

Dr. Grace H. Newell

NATRUM MURIATICUM: Isn't it curious how some physicians will hoot at a potency and fly like a frightened crow from a bacillus varying in size from 0.004 m.m. to 0.006 m.m. They can hardly eat, drink or sleep for fear a little microbe of the fifteenth culture will light on them somewhere, but there is nothing in a potency above the 12th.

Dr. E.B. Nash

PODOPHYLLUM PELTATUM: In the first onset of the disease, as well as in the very far advanced and apparently hopeless cases of cholera infantum, the 1000th potency (B. & T.) has done the best for me.

Dr. E.B. Nash

PULSATILLA: Don't pour down mother tincture of Pulsatilla by the 10 drop doses, as is the manner of those who do not believe in potentized remedies. You may give Pulsatilla in the high, higher, and highest potencies, and confidently expect the best results. I have often seen the delayed menses of young girls of Pulsatilla temperament appear promptly and naturally under the Materia Medica of Swan and cm. of Fincke (also with Kali carbonicum, Tuberculinum, and others).

Dr. E.B. Nash

RHUS TOX: I have used it both high and low, and find it useful all along the scale, but I have an m.m. potency made upon my own potentizer which has served me so well, and so many times, that I cannot refrain from speaking of it.

Dr. E.B. Nash

SECALE CORNUTUM: All the toes were attacked with dry gangrene. A few doses of Secale (high) afforded great relief, and checked the progress of the disease for a long time.

Dr. E.B. Nash

SELENIUM: Bad effects from drinking too much tea; all complaints are aggravated by it. Irresistible longing for spirituous liquors. Hoarseness, must often clear the throat of mucus especially at the beginning of singing. Irresistible desire for stimulants, wants to get drunk but feels worse after it. Very forgetful in business, but during sleep dreams of what he had forgotten. I have never used this metal below 200th potency.

Dr. E.B. Nash

SARSAPARILLA: Sarsaparilla is one of the best remedies for headache or periosteal pains generally, from suppressed gonorrhoea. I have seen great results from the 200th potency.

Dr. E.B. Nash

SPONGIA TOSTA: I live in a croupy climate and district, and after experimenting for 30 years, first with the low, then with the higher preparations, affirm that the 200th potency of this remedy does better work in croup than the lower preparations.

Dr. E.B. Nash

Sulphur: in cm. potency is generally efficacious in the case of ganglion.

Dr. J.H. Clarke

Those who use the potentized Sulphur can ever know what it is capable of curing.

Dr. E.B. Nash

The use of Thyroidin in 30 or 200 dilution will not only prevent grey hair but help in restoring natural colour. Give 30 for one month daily there after 200 every week for one month.

Dr. R.S. Das

14. GENERAL

ANTIMONIUM TARTARICUM: Now-a-days, washing out the stomach by lavage, and the rectum and colon by enemas, according to "Hall's method," is quite fashionable, and is withal much more sensible, inasmuch as they are so lame in their therapeutics.

Dr. E.B. Nash

ANTIMONIUM TARTARICUM: Notwithstanding these improvements, there is still a great deal of "gut scraping" going on in the name of "cleaning out the system," as though the alimentary canal was not a self-cleaning institution, if kept, or put into a healthy condition, but must be regularly "gone through" once in about so often, on the "house cleaning" principle.

Dr. E.B. Nash

ANTIMONIUM TARTARICUM: With Tartar emetic the face is always pale, or cyanotic, with no redness, and the breathing is not stertorous.

Dr. E.B. Nash

ANTIMONIUM TARTARICUM: It is also one of our best remedies for hepatization of lungs remaining after pneumonia. There is dullness on percussion, and lack, or absence of respiratory murmur, and shortness of breath, and patient continues pale, weak and sleepy.

Dr. E.B. Nash

Remedies only partly related to the case will change the character of the sickness so that no one can cure the case.

Dr. J.T. Kent

BAPTISIA TINCTORIA: Typhoid fever can be aborted under proper homoeopathic treatment, no matter what the old school says to the contrary.

Dr. E.B. Nash

BENZOIC ACID: Both Benzoic acid and Berberis are great remedies for arthritic troubles with the urinary symptoms.

Dr. E.B. Nash

BENZOIC ACID: In dribbling of urine of old men with enlarged prostate it has also done good service. The urine in the clothing scents the whole room.

Dr. E.B. Nash

BISMUTH: It is also often of benefit in cancer of the stomach, when there is at times vomiting of enormous quantities of food that seems to have lain in the stomach for days.

Dr. E.B. Nash

BORAX VENETA: It has also white, albuminous, starchy leucorrhoea, quite profuse, and with a sensation of warm water running down.

Dr. E.B. Nash

For the neuralgic pains (after operation on the eye) which often occur within the first 24 hours, relief can frequently be obtained from 5 drop doses of the tincture of Allium cepa.

Dr. Norton

CALCAREA OSTREARUM: Hering's advice when he says

'Treat the patient, not the disease."

Dr. E.B. Nash

CALCAREA PHOSPHORICA: Diarrhoea is very prominent, and the stools are green and "spluttering;" that is the flatulence (of which there is much) with the stool makes a loud spluttering noise when the stool passes.

Dr. E.B. Nash

CHAMOMILLA MATRICARIA: We might draw lines of differentiation between this and other restless remedies, but it would take too long. Each physician must get a habit of doing this for himself. In this ability to do this lies the superior skillfulness of the homoeopathic practitioner.

Dr. E.B. Nash

CAUSTICUM: On the other hand, it has all grades of nervous twitchings, chorea, convulsions and epileptic attacks, even progressive locomotor ataxia.

Dr. E.B. Nash

CAUSTICUM: Painful stiffness of the back and sacrum, especially on rising from a chair.

Dr. E.B. Nash

You can never definitely determine the power of the potentised remedy, but you should be able to realise when it is exhaused and its further application futile.

Dr. Boger

BELLIS PERENNIS: It is a grand friend to commerical travellers and railway spine of moderate severity, it has not any equal so for as my knowledge reaches. I think stasis lies at the bottom of these ailings.

Dr. Burnett

Cinchona Rubra and **Gention Q** in combination, 10 drops to be taken before meals, is an appetiser.

Dr. Ellis Barker

ARGENTUM NITRICUM: "I do believe that there is no need of cauterization with it except in the gonorrhoeal form of purulent conjunctivitis." Such testimony from such sources ought to shame the abuse of this agent in the hands of old school physicians, and sometimes bogus homoeopaths. In ophthalmia neonatorum in my own practice as a general practitioner I have had very often better success with Mercurius solubilis, especially where there was much purulent matter pouring out on opening the eyes.

Dr. A.B. Norton

It is seldom that the drug homoeopathically choosen fails to relieve insomnia. If there are no clear indications, Passiflora Q and Avena sat. Q in doses from 3 to 5 or more drops are useful aids and do not establish any drug habit.

Dr. Ruddock

A glass of cold water on rising in the morning with a level teaspoon of common table salt makes an excellent laxative.

Dr. Wheeler

DIOSCOREA VILL: 15 drops of tincture in hot water will

cause the intense pain of Appenticitis to fade away and give case to the patient.

Dr. Anchutz

DULCAMARA: It is quite a profitable business for one who has not much conscience and not much intelligence. But a conscientious physician feels worried and known he is not doing what he ought to do by his patient, unless he reaches out for the remedy which touches the constitution. It is far more useful to keep people from taking colds than to cure colds.

Dr. J.T. Kent

You do not get the full benefit of Homoeopathy and you cannot stop his stimulants because weakness will follow. Persons who have not taken wine as a regular beverage can and should do without it, as it interferes with the action of the homoeopathic remedy.

Dr. J.T. Kent

Healthy bile dissolves gall stones in the sac; healthy urine does the same to a stone in the pelvis of the kidney.

Dr. J.T. Kent

GELSEMIUM NITIDUM: One author says that Gelsemium stands midway between Aconite and Veratrum viride. I should rather place it between Baptisia and Belladonna.

Dr. E.B. Nash

GELSEMIUM NITIDUM: It is useful in the remittent fever of children. The fever is never of that active or violent form calling for Aconite or Belladonna, but of a milder form. The child lies drowsy, does not want to move, or, if it does, cannot move much on account of the weakness.

Dr. E.B. Nash

For the production of sleep, no remedy compares with Hyoscyamus in tincture 5 to 10 drops in half a glass of water and teaspoonful doses given half hourly.

Dr. Butler

KALI CARBONICUM: No remedy should ever be given on one symptom. If you are led to a remedy by a peculiar symptom, study the remedy and the disease thoroughly to as certain if the two are similar enough to each other to expect a cure. Any deviation from that rule is ruinous and will lead to the practice of giving medicines on single symptom.

Dr. J.T. Kent

KALI CARBONICUM: There are plenty of short acting remedies that would relieve the pain speedily, and at the close of the attack the constitutional remedy could then be given. If the patient can bear the pain to the end, it is better to wait until it passes off without any medicine. That sometimes is cruel, and then the short acting medicines should be given.

Dr. J.T. Kent

KALMIA LATIFOLIA: All the organs are related to each other, but especially the heart and kidneys. When the kidneys are not working well, the heart is very often troubles-one. All through the varying forms of Bright's disease the heart is troublesome. Difficulties of breathing, difficult heart action, with albuminuria. It will relieve the breathing. Again, associated with kidney affections, we have many eye complaints, difficulties of vision, and these also especially call for this remedy. It is often indicated in Bright's disease, with disturbance of vision, occurring during pregnancy.

Dr. J.T. Kent

KREOSOTUM: The case with the lochia after confinement, when the choice may lie between these three remedies, Kreosote, Rhus tox. and Sulphur. The other symptoms must decide between them. This ulceration may be found in cancer of the uterus, and then Kreosote will often be of great value. I have no doubt that many cases which degenerate into cancer might be prevented by its timely use. In some cases there is awful burning in the pelvis, as of red-hot coals, with discharge of clots in foul smelling blood. I see that Guernsey recommends it in cancer of the mammae, saying it is hard, bluish-red and covered with scurvy protuberances. I have never so used it, but in corrosive leucorrhoeas and ulcerations I have with great satisfaction. I generally use it in the 200th, with simply tepid water injections for cleanliness.

Dr. J.T. Kent

For burns stove or matches, quick dosing in cold water seems to promote faster pain relief and faster healing.

Dr. King

LACHESIS: You do not get all these things in the text, you have to see them applied, but the things I give you that are brought out clinically are those thing that have come from applying the symptoms of the remedy at the bed side to sick folks.

Dr. J.T. Kent

LACHESIS: It is seldom that you will see Lachesis headaches without cardiac difficulty.

Dr. J.T. Kent

LACHESIS: The symptoms of Lachesis have sometimes to be taken years after.

Dr. J.T. Kent

LEDUM PAL: The sides of a cut must be drawn togethers, and if it is perfectly tight it will heal itself by first intention. If it does not, then you may know there is a constitutional conditon that you must ferret out and find the remedy for. Local treatment must then be suspended. These remedies that I have mentioned, to a great extent, cover the management if wounds, and it is simple. Anyone has sense enough to draw together and close up a yawning wound, and to properly dress it. The muscles that naturally draw a wound open have to be overcome by stitching or by strappings. They do not belong to prescribing, they belong to the surgeon.

Dr. J.T. Kent

LEDUM PAL: Air is an irritant to a raw part and will keep up an unnecessary discharge of pus, even from a perfectly healthy sore.

Dr. J.T. Kent

MURIATIC ACID: There is decomposition of fluids; the stools are involuntary while passing urine; stools dark, thin, or haemorrhage of dark liquid blood. Mouth full of dark-bluish ulcers; unconscious. Moaning and sliding down in the bed from excessive weakness; lower jaw fallen, tongue dry, leathery and shrunken to a third of its natural size, and paralyzed; pulse weak and intermittent. It is hardly possible to draw a picture of a more desperate case of typhoid than this.

Dr. E.B. Nash

MAGNESIA PHOSPHORICA: I have no faith in the Schuesslerian theory in regard to it. Similia similibus curantur has stood the test with other remedies and will with the so-called tissues remedies regardless of theories.

Dr. E.B. Nash

MEDORRHINUM: The most characteristic difference between them is that with Medorrhinum the pains are worse in the day-time, and with Syphilinum in the night.

Dr. E.B. Nash

NATRUM MURIATICUM: We owe no obedience to man, not even to our parents, after we are old enough to think for ourselves. We owe obedience to truth.

Dr. J.T. Kent

NATRUM MURIATICUM: It not only removes the tendency to intermittent, but restores the patient to health, and takes away the tendency to colds—the susceptibility to colds, and to periodicity. It is the susceptibility that is removed. We know that every attack predisposes to another attack. Each attack of ague is move destructive than the previous one. The drugs used increase the susceptibility; the homoeopathic remedy removes the susceptibility. Homoeopathic treatment tends to simplify the human economy and to make disease more easily managed. Unless this susceptibility be eradicated, man goes down lower and lower into emaciation from above downwards.

Dr. J.T. Kent

NATRUM MURIATICUM: In dropsy after the malaria Natrum mur., when it acts curatively, generally brings back the original chill. The only cure known to man is from above down, from within out, and in the reverse order of coming. When it is otherwise, there is only improvement, not cure. When the symptoms return there is hope; that is the road to cure and there is no other.

Dr. J.T. Kent

NATRUM MURIATICUM: The homoeopathic failures are the worst failures on earth.

Dr. J.T. Kent

NATRUM MUR: Experienced physicians learn to classify patients by appearance.

Dr. J.T. Kent

NAJA TRIPUDIANS: There seems to be everything existing in one kingdom that exists in another. Then lowest is the mineral, the next the vegetable, and last the animal kingdom. If we had a perfect knowledge of anyone kingdom, we could probably cover the entire scope of curative possiblilities. But we have only a knowledge of a few remedies in each kingdom.

Dr. J.T. Kent

NAJA TRIPUDIANS: Another idea has been advanced that in any particular region, the vegetable kingdom provides all that is necessary for curing in that region.

Dr. J.T. Kent

NATRUM MURIATICUM: Examine every organ, not by examining it physically, for results of diseases do not led to the remedy, but examine the symptoms.

Dr. J.T. Kent

NATRUM MURIATICUM: Be sure that the remedy has not only the group of symptoms, but also the nature of the case.

Dr. J.T. Kent

NATRUM MURIATICUM: Map tongue is found under Natrum mur., Arsenicum alb., Lachesis, Nitric acid, and Taraxacum.

Dr. E.B. Nash

NATRUM CARBONICUM: Weakness of the ankles from childhood finds a good remedy in Natrum carb.

Dr. E.B. Nash

NITRIC ACID: The action of this remedy is just as positive upon the other outlet of the alimentary canal.

Dr. E.B. Nash

NATRUM SULPHURICUM: In chronic diarrhoea there is almost always some trouble with the liver, evidenced by soreness in right hypochondrium which is sensitive to touch, and hurts on walking or any jar.

Dr. E.B. Nash

NATRUM MURIATICUM: If the upper lip is much thickened or swollen, not of an erysipelatous character, we

.9

would think of three remedies, all of which have it, Belladonna, Calcarea ost., Natrum mur.

Dr. E.B. Nash

OPIUM: Everywhere opium is a producer of insensibility and partial or complete paralysis and, other things being equal, is homoeopthically indicated there.

Dr. E.B. Nash

PYROGEN: So far as prejudice against using such remedies is concerned, we should be an honest as was James B. Bell. when he said of Psorinum, "Whether derived from purest gold or purest filth, our gratitude for its excellent services forbids us to enquire or care."

Dr. E.B. Nash

PHOSPHORIC ACID: It is sin to keep such young people bowing down to hard study, and while it is true that youth is the time to get an education it is also true that it is the time when too great a strain in that direction may utterly wreck and forever incapacitate a mind which might, with more time and care, have been a blessing to the world.

Dr. E.B. Nash

Inter-costal Rheumatism yields for more quickly to Rananculus bulb. than to any other. (Aconite, Arnica, Bryonia.)

Dr. E.A. Farrington

Syzygium Q and **Uranium Nit. 3x** both combined or one after the other t.d.s. reduce the sugar in the urine in a fort-night.

Dr. Ghosal

SABADILLA: Prescribe for the patient first. No results of disease should be removed until proper constitutional treatment has been restorted to, and be sure that it is proper.

Dr. J.T. Kent

All substances absued as food become great remedies, such as vinegar, coffea, common salt, etc. We should look to them oftener than we do for the stubborn chronic cases.

Dr. J.T. Kent

STICTA PULMONARIA: I have found Sticta promptly curative in inflammatory rheumatism of the knee joint. It is very sudden in its attacks, and unless promptly relieved by Sticta will go on to the exudative stage and become chronic in character.

Dr. E.B. Nash

STICTA PULMONARIA: I have relieved many cases of chronic catarrh with Sticta; some of years' standing.

Dr. E.B. Nash

STAPHISAGRIA: It is one of the best for affections of the prostate gland in old men, with frequent unrination and dribbling of urine afterwards.

Dr. E.B. Nash

SPONGIA TOSTA: The cough is dry and sibilant, or sounds like a saw driven through a pine board, each cough corresponding to a thrust of the saw. Croup often comes on after exposure to dry, cold winds. It generally comes on in the evening, with high fever, excitement and fearfulness.

Dr. E.B. Nash

THUJA OCCIDENTALIS: Finally don't forget to look for the three miasms in all obstinate cases, whether acute or chronic.

Dr. E.B. Nash

It is very seldom that fear will give a man inflammation, but fear is a common cause of inflammation of the uterus, and of the ovaries, in plethoric, vigorous, exitable woman.

Dr. J.T. Kent

In biliary colic, Calcarea carb. has never failed me.

Dr. Hughes

15. SPECIAL POINTERS
OF
SOME REMEDIES

ANTIMONIUM CRUDUM: "Copious haemorrhage from the bowels, mixed with solid faces; chronic redness of the eyelids; toothache in decayed teeth, worse at night; gastric trouble after acids, sour wine, vinegar," etc.

Dr. E.B. Nash

ACONITUM NAPELLUS: There is no better picture in a few words of the Aconite fever than is given by Hering-"Heat, with thirst; hard, full and frequent pulse, anxious impatience, inappeasable, beside himself, tossing about with agony."

Dr. E.B. Nash

ARSENICUM ALBUM: In every one of these affections, ranging along the whole length of the anal, and from the lightest grade of irritation to the most intense inflammatory and malignant forms of disease, we will be apt to find everywhere present the characteristic burning of this remedy, in greater or lesser degree; and the not less characteristic amelioration from heat, and also, though not quite so invariably, the midnight aggravation.

Dr. E.B. Nash

ARSENICUM patient is weak out of proporation to the rest of his trouble.

Dr. E.B. Nash

ALUMINA is one of the best remedies for haemorrhages of the bowels in typhoid fever.

Dr. E.B. Nash

ANTIMONIUM TARTARICUM: The nausea of this remedy is an intense as that of Ipecacuanha, but not so persistent, and there is relief after vomiting. I have found it nearest a specific (of course we know there is no absolute specific for any disease) for cholera morbus of any remedy. For more than 25 years, I have seldom found it necessary to use any other, and then only when there were severe cramps in the stomach and bowels, when Cuprum metallicum relieved.

Dr. E.B. Nash

ANTIMONIUM TART: If Antimonium tart. possessed only the one power of curing that it does upon the respiratory organs, it would be indispensable. No matter what the name of the trouble, whether it be bronchitis, pneumonia, whooping cough or asthma, if there is great accumulation of mucus with coarse rattling, of filling up with it, but, at the same time, there seems to be inability to raise it, Tartar emetic is the first remedy to be thought of. This is true in all ages and constitutions, but particularly so in children and old people.

Dr. E.B. Nash

ARGENTUM NITRICUM: Guernsey says, "We think of this remedy on seeing a withered and dried up person, made so by disease." This especially in children. "He looks like a little withered old man." (Fluoric acid, young people look old) Argentum like gold profoundly affects the mind.

Dr. E.B. Nash

ARGENTUM NITRICUM: Also in epilepsy or convulsions; in the former (epilepsy) one characteristic symptom is that for hours or days before the attack the pupils are dilated; in the latter the convulsions are preceded for a short time by great restlessness.

Dr. E.B. Nash

ARGENTUM NITRICUM: In blepharitis Graphites and Staphisagria have served me oftener than Argentum nitricum.

Dr. E.B. Nash

ANTIMONIUM CRUDUM: It is especially to be considered if the gastric derangement is of recent date. The process of digestion is hardly under way; the eructations taste of the food as he ate it, and the sufferer feels as if he must "throw up" before there will be any relief. In such a case a few pellets of Antimonium crudum on the tongue will often settle the business, save the loss of a meal, and all further suffering.

Dr. E.B. Nash

ARSENICUM ALBUM: I do not think this is sound reasoning or good advice, for I have never found any rule by which I could decide from the beginning that a case would later on develop into a case of the pernicious or malignant character which would ever call for the exhibition of Arsenic.

Dr. E.B. Nash

Arsenicum alb. is of great service in epithelioma (Cancer) of the nose and lips.

Dr. J.T. Kent

ARGENTUM NITRICUM: "Pain in the back (small of) relieved when standing or walking, but severe when rising from a seat," is a condition often found in practice. I have often relieved it with Sulphur or Causticum, but remember also Argentum nitricum.

Dr. E.B. Nash

APIS acts on the synovial membranes, giving a perfect picture of synovitis, particularly when it affects the knee.

Dr. E.A. Farrington

Arsenicum is an excellent remedy for baldness, if the hair fall out in consequence of an impoverished condition of the follicles, the scalp and the skin generally are dry, and the patients assimilative powers are impaired.

Dr. Charles Hempel

There are few remedies in the entire Materia Medica having impaired memory as so marked a characteristic. In restoring the memory Anacard cures the patient of all other troubles.

Dr. Guernsey

Arthritis Deformans responds to Antimonium crudum—a near specific.

Dr. Schwarts

Argentum nitricum cures Claustro-phobia.

Dr. M.L. Tyler

The strong tincture of Arnica applied to wasp sting presents the pain, and swelling, and in a couple of hours, the sting is forgotten.

Dr. M.L. Tyler

In true carditis, pericarditis, Aconite 30 in watery solution; generally accomplishes everything that can be desired.

Dr. Jahr

In Cancrum oris and severe forms of aphthac and generally in malignant inflammations and phagedenic conditions of the parts, Arsenicum has no rival.

Dr. Hering

In the form of diarrhoea oftenest with old people, which alternates with constipation, Antimonium crudum is the only remedy.

Dr. M.L. Tyler

Sleeplessness caused by over-exertion and extreme weariness of mind or body. Here Arnica never fails to summon the tired. Natures sweet restorer balmy sleep.

Dr. M.L. Tyler

We have no remedy which equals Arnica in concussion of brain or spine or both.

Dr. E.A. Farrington

Arsenicum is the remedy for debility resulting from over taxing of the muscular tissues, such as follows prolonged exertion, climbing mountains etc.

Dr. E.A. Farrington

Arnica should be administered whenever there is muscular fatigue from whatever cause. Its power to aid the restoration of exhausted muscle is truely wonderful.

Dr. Ruddock

Judging from our own experience, in the debility of cancer, Hydrastis must yield palm to Arsenicum, for we have repeatedly witnessed the most decided improvement from a course of Arsenicum.

Dr. Ruddock

Aloe 6th dilution is reported to have cured falling of hair.

Dr. Ruddock

If you find a mydriasis on the left side, this should make you look for Anacardium.

Dr. Med. Milar Deichmann

Dr. Roger in his little synoptic key, gives three remedies for nail biting; Arsenic, Sanicula and Hyoscyamus. I have found **Sanicula** to be the most effective in treating that condition.

Dr. Dixon

Adrenalinum 200 to 10M gives me great results in what other doctors pronounce high pressure and its results.

Dr. W.A. Yingling

Arsenicum is suitable in every form, the mildest to the most severe.

Dr. Boehr

I think nail biting was due to some nervous irritation. Ammonium bromatum is the remedy in the repertory for nail biting. It is the only one there and I think it works.

Dr. Gier

Ammonium carb. has bleeding from intestines with each monthly period.

Dr. Leon Vannier

Leutic headaches, especially the nocturnal react well the Aurum and above all to Aurum iodatum.

Dr. Donnar

Blisers on the hands from heavy manual labour disappear overnight after the application of 10% Aristolochia ointment.

Dr. Julius Mezger

Ordinary lumbago yielde of the very readily to the internal and external use of Aconite.

Dr. Hempel

BRYONIA: With Bryonia it is excessive dryness or lack of secretion in them. It begins in the lips, which are parched, dry and cracked, and only ends with the rectum and stools, which are hard and dry as if burnt.

Dr. E.B. Nash

BRYONIA: It makes no difference what the name of the disease, if the patient feels greatly, > by lying still and suffers greatly on the slightest motion, and the more and longer he moves the more he suffers, Bryonia is the first remedy to be thought of, and there must be very strong counter-indications along other lines that will rule it out.

Dr. E.B. Nash

BRYONIA: The characteristic pains of inflammatory affections of the serous membranes are stitching pains; this is the reason why Bryonia comes to be such a renal remedy in pleuritis, meningitis, peritonitis, pericarditis, etc. The subjective symptoms corresponding to the remedy must go down before it, and the objectives must as surely follow.

Dr. E.B. Nash

BERBERIS VULGARIS: No matter what ails the patient, if he has persistent pain as above described in the region of the kidneys do not forget Berberis.

Dr. E.B. Nash

The more Benzoic acid is used in gout, the more it will be prized.

Dr. C. Hering

BELLADONNA: No remedy has greater affinity for the throat. The burning, dryness (Sabadilla), sense of constriction (constant desire to swallow to relieve the sense of dryness, Lyssin), with or without swelling of the palate and tonsils, is sometimes intense. I once witnessed a case of poisoning in which these symptoms were terribly distressing.

Dr. E.B. Nash

BISMUTH: The surface is warm and often covered with warm sweat. The face is deathly pale, with rings around the eyes. This is a perfect picture of Bismuth, and no other remedy need be confounded with it.

Dr. E.B. Nash

BERBERIS VULGARIS: It is especially to be thought of in arthritic and rheumatic affections, when these back symptoms, connected with urinary alterations are present. One very characteristic symptom is a bubbling sensation in the region of the kidneys. Another is soreness in region of kidneys when jumping out of a wagon or stepping hard downstairs or from any jarring movement.

Dr. E.B. Nash

I have myself frequently obtained much reduction in the size of the ganglion situated at the back of the wrist by the external application of Benzoic acid in an ointment.

Dr. Hughes

In the giddiness of elderly people (cerebral stasis), Bellis peren., acts well and does permanent good.

Dr. Burnott

If you ever get a case of sea sickness and you are in doubt between Petroleum and Tabacum, which is the other common drug for sea sickness, you almost always get that occipital headache as well as the sea sickness in Petroleum, and Tabacum people have not.

Borax acts in the majority of cases of air sickness, because it is sudden dip which upsets most people, and particularly their terror of falling. I have had a number of cases in which I have completely stopped air sickness by 3 or 4 doses of Borax before they started flying.

Dr. D.M. Borland

An inter-current course of Bacillinum will often make wonderful charge in patient who have a personal or family history of chest affections.

Dr. J.H. Clarks

Baccilus Morgan has removed superficial congestive swellings of the hands and feet where no definite pathology would account for it.

Dr. William B. Griggs

CARBO VEGETABILIS: Coldness or the knees, even in bed (Apis); of left arm and left leg; very cold hands and feet; fingernails blue.

Dr. E.B. Nash

CALCAREA OSTREARUM: Sensations of coldness in single parts should always call to mind Calcarea, as well as general coldness. (Cistus and Heloderma.)

Dr. E.B. Nash

CHAMOMILLA MATRICARIA: In the Chamomilla case the patient is exceedingly sensitive to the pain and exclaims continually, "Oh; I cannot bear the pain." Many times have I met this condition in labor cases, and in the majority of them the cross, peevish snappish, condition of mind accompenying, and seen it changed in a short time to a mild, uncomplaining, patient state, by a single dose of Chamomilla 200th.

Dr. E.B. Nash

CHAMOMILLA MATRICARIA: It was in my earlier practice, when I was prescribing for names more than I do now, and of course he got Aconite, Bryonia and Rhus toxicodendron, etc., but no relief. A wiser man was called in consultation and the patient was quickly cured by Chamomilla. When I asked the counsel what led him to prescribe this remedy he answered numbness with the pains.

Dr. E.B. Nash

COFFEA CRUDA: Hering used to recommend Aconite and Coffea in alternation in painful inflammatory affections, where the fever symptoms of the former and also the nervous sensibility of the latter were present, and I know of no two remedies that alternate better, though I never do it, since I learned to closely individualize.

Dr. E.B. Nash

CUPRUM METALLICUM: Dunham said, "In Camphor collapse is most prominent; in Veratrum album, the evacuation and vomiting; in Cuprum, the cramps."

Dr. E.B. Nash

CAUSTICUM: Causticum also has very marked action upon the urinary organs, as is shown by the following symptoms; "Itching of the orifice of the urethra." "Constant ineffectual desire to urinate, frequent evacuations of only a few drops, with spasms in the rectum and constipation."

This is like Nux vomica and Cantharis, and I once cured a chronic case of cystitis in a married woman, which had baffled the best efforts of several old school physicians, eminent for their skill, for years.

Dr. E.B. Nash

CAUSTICUM: "He urinates so easily that he is not sensible of the stream, and scarcely believes in the dark that he is urinating at all, until he make sure by sence of touch."

Dr. E.B. Nash

CAUSTICUM: In influenza or what is now called La Grippe it disputes for first place with Eupatorium perf. and Rhus toxid. All three have a tired, sore, bruised sensation all over the body, and all have soreness in the chest when coughing, but if involuntary micturition is present Causticum wins.

Dr. E.B. Nash

CAUSTICUM: No homoeopath can afford to be without an understanding of Causticum upon the respiratory organs.

Dr. E.B. Nash

CHELIDONIUM MAJUS: If we should find pressive pain in the region of the liver, whether it be enlarged and sensitive to pressure or not, bitter taste in the mouth, togue coated thickly yellow, with red margins showing imprint of the teeth, yellowness of whites of eyes, face, hands and skin; stools gray, clay coloured, or yellow as gold, urine also yellow as gold, lemon coloured or dark brown, leaving a yellow colour on vessel when emptied out, loss of appetite, disgust and nausea, or vomiting of bilious matter, and especially if patient could retain nothing but hot drinks on the stomach, we would have a clear case for Chelidonium even though the infra-scapular pain were absent. All these symptoms might be found in either a chronic or acute case.

Dr. E.B. Nash

CALCAREA PHOSPHORICA: The Phosphorus element in this preparation seems to change the temperament, for while it retains its wonderful remedial power over tardy bone development it acts best in spare subjects instead of fat. So that if we find a sickly child with fontanelles remaining open too long or re-opening after once closed, the child being spare and anaemic, we think of this remedy.

Dr. E.B. Nash

CARBO ANIMALIS: The subjects of it are often disposed to glandular swellings, indurations and suppurations.

Dr. E.B. Nash

Cannabis Indica should be remembered if we ever come across a case of catalepsy. In its power of causing catalepsy, its only rival is the chloride of tin.

Dr. Hughes

CHOLELIGHIASIS: The remedy to cure the condition parmanently is Cinchona. (Continue it for a number of months.)

Dr. E.A. Ferrington

There is one point of practical importance according to my own opinion, with regard to Bryonia, namely that supposing Aconite had not preceded it in the treatment of Bronchitis and also in the treatment of Acute Rheumatism, I have almost invariably found that Bryonia does not begin to produce its curative action until a few doses of Aconite have been first administered.

Dr. Hale

10

Patients who come to hospital complaining of severe cramps, especially in calves very often have to get either Cuprum or Calcarea.

Dr. M.L. Tyler

If a case seems to be Pulsatilla, but the mental state is peevish and irritable, rather than mild, try Cyclamen. It will often work wonders.

Homoeo. Recorder, Aug. 31

I have repeatedly killed tape worm with Cina as well as the lumbrici and ascarides.

Dr. Bayes

Dreamy state, indifference to disease, and even death; absence of efforts to get well, absence of interest in the present, utter complacency to future and drowsy state indicates Clematis arecto flora.

Dr. Hughes

Many cases of rheumatoid arthritis in women begin at the manopause whenever this is the case and the small joints of hands and feet are involved, Caulophyllum should be one of the drugs; also in any non-menopausal cases where uterus and small joints are affected.

Dr. M.L. Tyler

Homoeopathy knows no specifics except the specific remedy for the individual, yet, as Hahnemann teaches us, some remdies so exactly reproducs a diseased condition, as to become specific. Such are Cantharis in systilis, Belladonna in scarlet fever, Merc. cor. in dysentery and Latro. m., in angina pectoris.

Dr. M.L. Tyler

Cantharis internally in homoeopathic potency, is a very old tip for charming away the pains of burns.

Dr. M.L. Tyler

Remember the use of Coffea for fatigue arising from long journeys, especially during hot weather.

Dr. E.A. Farrington

In the form of ordinary Camphor pilules, I have found it an excellent remedy in simple sleeplessness.

Dr. J.H. Clarke

Calcarea carb. for deep abscesses. These will get absorbed or become Calcareous.

Dr. A.N. Mukherji

According to the experience of others and my own Caladium is the most efficient remedy Pruritus valval.

Dr. C.G. Raue

Coffea will remove the severest pains which drive the patients almost frantic; they cry, tremble, do not know what to do; the pain is indiscribable; it is momentarily relieved by holding cold water in mouth.

Dr. C.G. Raue

CARBO VEGETABILIS often at the drink of death a saviour in those state of collapse, dissolution of blood and paralytic conditions, which seem rapidly to involve the whole organism.

Dr. C.G. Raue

CANTHARIS will relieve the raw burning pain and promotes healing; covers acute nephritis which may ensure.

Dr. Charles C. Boericke

A drenaline China 200 gave dramatic relief in acute bronchial asthma and 1M also palliates, but Arsenicum alb., to be followed for weakness.

Homoeo. Recorder Feb., 24

Use Cadmium phosphate in suspected carcinoma of prostate.

Dr. Wilbur K. Bond

In lingering remittent fevers of children, having symptoms of helminthiasis with or without worms, Cina is specific.

Dr. Chepmall

Cannabis Indica is the most useful medicine we possess for diminishing the frequency of the paroxysms of migraine.

Dr. Ringer

DIGITALIS PURPUREA: The only tonic, in the sense of something to impart strength or tone to the human organism, is nourishing food.

Dr. E.B. Nash

DROSERA can be used as a pathological remedy for Tubercular glands.

Dr. M.L. Tyler

In Drosera gland cases, one notices not only the diminution in the size of the gland, but that the old scars fade away, get free and come to the surface, that discolouration goes, and that when a gland does break down under Drosera, it behaves in a very restrained manner, with a small opening, little discharge and that it leaves practically nothing to mark what has taken place.

Dr. M.L. Tyler

Euphrasia has a shining face which looks as if it had been varnished, the skin of the face cracks as varnish does. The face feels stiff.

Dr. H.A. Roberts

PERRUM METALLICUM: It is true that when iron is introduced into the system in large quantities with a view to supplying a deficiency of iron in the blood that it is not assimilated, but may be almost entirely obtained from the faeces, having been eliminated by the intestines.

Dr. E.B. Nash

NATRUM MURIATICUM: I have seen better cures of bad cases of anaemia by Natrum muriaticum in potentized form than I ever did from Iron in any form, although Iron has its cases, as have also Pulsatilla, Cyclamen, Calcarea phos., Carbo veg., China and many other remedies.

Dr. E.B. Nash

GELSEMIUM NITIDUM: One notable characteristic is that

sometimes the headache is relieved by a profuse flow of urine. (Lac defloratum has a profuse flow of urine during sick headache to which it is adapted, but the pain is not so markedly relieved by the flow.

Dr. E.B. Nash

No remedy can at all be compared with Gelsemium Q 1 to 5 drops every 30 minutes to produce relaxation of a rigid unyielding os-uteri in labour.

Dr. Douglas

HEPAR SULPHURIS: The Hepar asthma is worse in dry cold air and better in damp, while Natrum sulph. is exactly the opposite like Dulcamara. There is no other remedy that I know that has the amelioration so strongly in damp weather as Hepar sulphur.

Dr. E.B. Nash

Among the remedies for prevention of skin stroke, Gelsemium is the most important.

Dr. C.G. Raue

I should content, led by my own experience, that the Hydrastis treatment is the very best known for this dire disease. It improves the appetite and condition of the patient generally. Under its use, the complexion alters, the state of the blood improves. It marvellously allays the pain of cancer, in this respect altogether surpassing Opium; Morphia or any so-called anodyne. It retards the growth of cancer.

Dr. Gutteridge

The sick headaches of women, are a type of case in which

a nosode may be required. Although these headaches may be relieved by such remedies as Iris versicolor. they are not really cured by them, and have a tendency to recure with increasing severity. Such a condition may be permanently cured by Tuberculinum in high potency, administered at infrequent intervals in between the acute attacks.

Dr. Nemo

IPECACUANHA: The spasmodic cough and asthma do not seem to all depend upon accumulation of mucus, for Ipecacuanha is often our best remedy in the first stage of both asthma and whooping cough, before the stage when the mucus is present.

Dr. E.B. Nash

KALI CARBONICUM: In what I have written I do not pretend to have told, all, and if I thought that any young physician would be led to rely alone upon this work of mine or be led away from thorough study of the Materia Medica instead of to it I would stop writing.

Dr. E.B. Nash

KALI HYDROIODICUM: A medicine which gradually induces a change in the habit or constitution, and restores healthy functions without sensible evacuation.

Dr. E.B. Nash

When you are struck with a Kali bich migraine that does not respond always remember Iris.

Dr. D.M. Borland

Dr. Logan reported the successful treatment of more than 200 cases of Diphtheria with Hydrastis gargle.

Dr. Ruddock

Kali mur.: is a well proven anti-infective and anti-virus remedy.

Dr. Koppikar

I found that the prolonged use of **Drosera** induces tuberculization in animals and its power to cure tuberculization never fails me.

Dr. Curie

Lachesis: Its action is perfectly homoeopathic to acute yellow atrophy of the liver.

Dr. Jausset

Loose Velt said that a half open condition of the eyes during sleep pointed to Lycopodium.

Dr. Sidwick

Rheumatism with constipation is a leading indication for Bach's intestinal nosode Bach Polyvalent 200.

Dr. Edward Whitmont

In taking your case and hunting through your repertories and Materia Medicas, don't make the mistake of getting a remedy too firmly fixed in your mind, or you court disaster.

Dr. Boger

Lycopodium can also be an intermediary remedy in cases

where the correctly selected remedies are no longer effective. Therefore Lycopodium is called the vegetable Sulphur.

Dr. Med. H. Zulla

In girls, Lycopodium is a remedy for Amenorrhoea, with non-development of breasts in such girls and makes the course appear.

Dr. Leon Renard

Lycopodium is particularly adopted to the treament of cirrhosis of the liver.

Dr. Boehr

I always give Lyssin for every dog bite. I have ever had, and I have never seen anything but the best of results-it relieves the pain and they never have any bad effects at all. They always heal up; as a routine proposition. I give Lyssin.

Dr. A.H. Grimmer

LACHESIS: Exceptional loquacity, with rapid change of subjects; jumps abruptly from one idea to another.

Dr. E.B. Nash

LACHESIS: Hempel wrote in his first volume of Materia Medica: "In spite of every effort to the contrary, the conviction has gradually forced itself upon my mind that the pretended pathogenesis of Lachesis, which has emanated from Dr. Hering's otherwise meritorius and highly praiseworthy efforts, is a great delusion, and that with the exception of the poisonous effects with which this publication is abundantly mingled the balance of the symptoms are unreliable."

Hempel modified his views somewhat, I think, in later editions.

Dr. E.B. Nash

LAC CANINUM: If the breasts and throat get sore during menstruation, especially if the menses flow in gushes instead of continuously, Lac caninum is the remedy.

Dr. E.B. Nash

LILIUM TIGRINUM: The uterine symptoms are sometimes marked so as to be over-looked for the time by the violence of the heart symptoms.

Dr. E.B. Nash

LYCOPODIUM has often saved neglected, mal-treated or imperfectly cured cases of pneumonia from running into consumption.

Dr. E.B. Nash

LYCOPODIUM: If you find corresponding failure in the sensorium of old men, the memory fails, they use wrong words to express themselves, mix things up generally in writing, spelling, and are, in short, unable to do ordinary mental work on account of failing brain power, remember Lycopodium.

Dr. E.B. Nash

LYCOPODIUM: A feeling of satiety is found under this remedy which alternates with a feeling of hunger of a peculiar kind.

Dr. E.B. Nash

LYCOPODIUM: The liver troubles of Lycopodium are more apt to be of the atrophic variety, while those of China are hypertrophic, both being equally useful in their sphere.

Lycopodium has almost, if not quite, as marked action upon the urinary organs as upon the liver.

Dr. E.B. Nash

MERCURIUS: No remedy has this condition of mouth in any degree equal to Mercury.

Dr. E.B. Nash

MERCURIUS: The glands and bones also come strongly under the influence of this remedy. The glandular swellings are cold, inclined to suppurate, having these chilly creepings forementioned. These with the bone-pains in the exostoses and caries are all aggravated at night in the warmth of the bed.

Dr. E.B. Nash

MERCURIUS: It must be remembered that Mercury is no more a panacea for syphilis than is Sulphur for psora or Thuja for sycosis, also there would be no truth in similia similibus.

Dr. E.B. Nash

MERCURIUS CORROSIVUS: It seems, according to the testimony of others, to be a useful remedy for catarrhal affections of the eyes and nose. Here also I have no testimony to offer, but would not cast doubt upon it for that reason. I do not desire to place my own experience ahead of that of others. We are co-laborers. Let each add to the general store of medical knowledge, that all may draw freely from it as oc⊾ sion demands.

Dr. E.B. Nash

For elongated uvula causing trouble, apply a little of low trituration of Mercurius Corrosivus on uvula, and it will relieve immediatly and permanently.

Dr. R.B. Das

Muriatic acid cures the muscular weakness following excessive use of Opium and tobacco. (Veratrum alb., Pulsatilla, Avena sativa, Ipecac.)

Dr. H.C. Allen

Dysmenorrhoea: Single dose of the Magnesia Phos., cm. just any time the patient happened to come up, not necessarily during the painful period, have cured for us quite a number of cases.

Dr. M.L. Tyler

I became convinced that filariasis should be treated as a Psora-Syphilitic disease and that Mercurius sulphuricus was the appropriate remedy. I tried the same remedy in cases of the same degrees of chronicity, utilising the several potencies of the remedy up to m.m. potency according to the nature of each case, and have suceeded in curing a very large number of cases. Though this amounts to routine practice, I consider this remedy as a specific for this particular disease, and this may be used safely in all cases. In the more chronic cases, though the swelling has continued for a long time, the parts have lost their hardness and became soft, and the patients have become free and normal in general health.

Dr. T.S. Iyer

The more frequent relapses sit in, the more specially is Mercurius indicated. (Acute rheumatism.)

Dr. Boehr

Morgan Bacillus is useful in arthritis where nothing else works.

Dr. Robert H. Farley

Mercurius is a specific remedy in a great number of cases of jaundice.

Dr. Laurie

Magnesia phos. can relieve the excruciating pain of cancer.

Dr. Heselton

NUX VOMICA: For instance, in Rhus the loose cough is worse in the morning, the tight, dry one in the evening.

Dr. E.B. Nash

NUX VOMICA: The pressure as from a stone occurs also under Bryonia and Pulsatilla.

Dr. E.B. Nash

NATRUM MURIATICUM: Natrum mur. also cures the headaches of school girls, and here it may be difficult to choose between it and Calcarea phos. both remedies also being particularly adapted to anaemic states. Indeed, I have sometimes missed and had to give Calcarea phos. when Natrum failed and vice versa, because I could not make the choice.

Dr. E.B. Nash

NATRUM MURIATICUM: Of course the intense thirst of salt is well known, and keeps pace with the hunger. Now this is the case with diabetes, for which Natrum is a curative if otherwise indicated. In all of these cases, of course, it must be used high, for we get the low in our food.

Dr. E.B. Nash

Saw Palmetto, besides its well written up action on the prostate gland, can now take its stand as a beautifying remedy, since it promotes in a marked degree the growth of the mammary gland in women.

Dr. Dewey

NATRUM SULPHURICUM: One point in the digestive upset of Natrum sulph. is that whether it is a gall bladder or liver upset or whether it is an Appendix, concurrently with the attack, the patients are liable to get a suppurative condition about the root of the nails. I have verified it several times. A patient with chronic liver who whenever he is getting a slight increase of disturbance, begins to develop suppurating places round his nails, will very often run to Naturm sulphuricum.

Dr. D.M. Borland

NATRUM MURIATICUM in brandy, a table-spoonful evenings, is said to produce conception, from intercourse the following night. Several surprising examples of this have been related to me.

Dr. Hering

If vertigo and headache be very persistent or prostration be prolonged after Natrum, Nux vomica will relieve.

Dr. H.C. Allen

In caps is recommended by Hahnemann for home-sickness with flushed cheeks, he has uttered a truth, the correctness of which every practitioner can easily verify if he chooses. (Ign., Phosphoric acid, Merc. sol.)

Dr. Jahr

Natrum carb. was sometimes very effective in cases which displayed very little reaction, especially in elderly people.

Dr. Alva Benjamin

OPIUM: I will say just here that any homoeopathic physician that feels obliged to use Opium or its alkaloid in this way and for this purpose does not understand his business and had better study his Materia Medica, and the principles of applying it according to Hahnemann, or else go over to the old school where they make no pretensions to have any law of cure. In the first place Opium in narcotic doses does not produce sleep, but stupor, and it only relieves pain by rendering the patient unconscious to it. How many cases have been so masked by such treatment, that the disease progressed until there was no chance fo cure? Pain, fever and all other symptoms are the voice of the disease, telling where is the trouble and guiding us to the remedy.

Dr. E.B. Nash

PULSATILLA: The bad taste in the mouth is persistent and the loss of taste is frequent, as is also the loss of smell.

Dr. E.B. Nash

PULSATILLA: The haemorrhages flow, and stop, and flow again; continually changing. the stools in diarrhoea constantly change in colour; they are green, yellow, white, watery or slimy; as Guernsey expresses it, "no two stools alike."

Dr. E.B. Nash

In homoeopathy, medicines can never replace each other nor be as good as another.

Dr. Kent, Dr. Hahnemann, Dr. Piere Schmidt

PHOSPHORIC ACID: Let us remember that the profound weakness and depression of Phosphoric acid is upon the sensorium and nervous system, and will be there whether diarrhoea is present or not. It is markedly so in typhoids, so I can fully attest from abundant observation.

Dr. E.B. Nash

PSORINUM: I have cured eruptions on the skin resembling itch with Psorinum, rheumatic troubles that were very obstinate under our usual remedies with Medorrhinum and a long standing case of caries of the spine with Syphilinum, but in not one of these cases had the patient, that I could trace, itch, gonorrhoea or syphilis.

Dr. E.B. Nash

PLUMBUM METALLICUM: H. Guernsey claimed great powers for it in jaundice; whites of eyes, skin, stool and urine all are very yellow, and I have prescribed it with success.

Dr. E.B. Nash

When a mother says, she has no milk or that the milk is scanty, thicker, unhealthy, dries up soon, Phytolacca becomes then a constitutional remedy if there are no contra indicating symptoms.

Dr. J.T. Kent

Phosphorus is the only remedy which never fails to cure pigeon chest; it should be given for a long time day at least three months during which time, the chest will be normal.

Dr. E.B. Nash

I have found at least several times that a remedy like Psorinum which is so terribly chilly, is necessary in the course of treatment of deep allergies, inspite of the fact that the patient is very warm blooded.

Dr. Schmidt

I find Phosphorus especially indicated in young men who are trying to restrain their natural sexual passion and yet there is locally erethism. This Phosphorus helps most wonderfully to control.

Dr. E.A. Farrington

Pyrogen is sometimes useful when there is a history of septicaemia, severe after effects of dental extraction, or ill-health commencing after an abortion, in the absence of any obvious pelvic pathology.

Dr. Foubister

In any psychoneurotic group of patients, there are those with present fatigue, worse in the morning, who say they feel more tired on arising than they went to bed, and also mention that the least desk work leaves them dragged out and listless I will now give more thought to Picric acid.

Dr. Robert L. Redfield

RHUS TOXICODENDRON: Great sensitiveness to open

11

air; putting the hand from under the bed cover brings on the cough (Bar., Hepar.)

Back; Pain between the shoulders on swallowing.

Cough during chill; dry, teasing, fatiguing, but urticaria over body during heat.

Dr. E.B. Nash

RHUS TOX: Indeed Rhus is one or our best remedies in lumbago.

Dr. E.B. Nash

RHUS TOX: Whenever in fevers or even inflammatory diseases the sensorium becomes cloudy (smoky) or stupefaction sets in, with low grade of muttering delirium, dry tongue, etc., we think of Rhus.

Dr. E.B. Nash

If a patient complains of rheumatic pains and with it there is present restlessness and inability to keep quiet, consider Trombidium before jumping to the conclusion that it is a Rhus tox. case.

Homoeo. Recorder, Jan. 31

Experience has shown that a vitaminitic troubles arising from eating too much cooked meat are best treated with Sulphur.

Dr. F.H. Bellokossy

All carcinomas I have to treat now who have had x-rays, I put on to one of the radio active salts as a first measure to try to antidote the x-rays. Usually I use one of the Radium salts—Radium mromide or Radium iodide. If I can find any indication for Iodine, I prefer the Radium Iodide, to Radium Bromide.

Dr. E.M. Borland

The specific remedy for lumbago is not Pulsatilla, as was formerly supposed, but Rhus tox. so far I have cured about every case that I have had to treat, with Rhus tox. in three to four days, except parhaps two or three cases where I had to complete the cure with Pulsatilla.

Dr. Jter

SULPHUR: I now come to an attempt to give some idea of the curative sphere of Hahnemann's king of anti-psorics. I do not in this place feel it incumbent upon me to enter into a defence of Hahnemann's psora theory against those who discard it because they do not understand it. With those who do understand and profit by it there is no need of such defence. The truth stands confirmed (with those who have put to the test Hahnemann's rules for the use of Sulphur) that it has power to mont and overcome certain obstacles to the usual action of drugs when indicated by the symptoms, or least seemingly so. That is the reason why the indication as laid down in the books reads; "When seemingly indicated drugs do not cure, use Sulphur," because psora is the obstacle to be oversome.

Dr. E.B. Nash

SULPHUR: Let no one understand that Sulphur is the only remedy capable of removing psoric complications, but simply that Sulphur will be likely to be oftener indicated here, because it oftener covers the usual manifestations of psora in its pathogenesis than any other remedy. There are anti-psorics, like Psorinum, Causticum, Graphites, etc., which may have to be used instead of Sulphur. And we know which one by the same law which guides us in the selection of the right remedy any time.

Dr. E.B. Nash

SULPHUR: There is one thing about Sulphur that is often underestimated by the profession in general, viz., its power of absorption. It is after the state of effusion has set in or even later when this stage is passed and the results of the inflammatory process are to be gotten rid of; like the enlargement of the joints in rheumatism, exudations into serous sacs, pleura, meningeal membranes, peritoneum, etc. Bryonia is one of the remedies first thought of in these cases, and we have another remedy that is making a record for itself here, viz., Kali muriaticum but when the case is complicated by psora and, especially, when the characteristic burnings stand out prominently Sulphur is almost sure to be needed before the case is finished.

Dr. E.B. Nash

SILICEA: Promotes expulsion of foreign bodies from the tissues, fish bones, needles, bone splinters.

Dr. E.B. Nash

SEPIA: A short walk fatigues her very much. She faints easily from extremes of cold or heat, after getting wet, from riding in a carriage, while kneeling at church, and on other trifling occasion.

Dr. E.B. Nash

SANGUINARIA CANADENSIS: Sometimes indicated

after Sulphur and Lachesis have failed, especially if the circumscribed redness of the cheeks appears.

Dr. E.B. Nash

SARSAPARILLA: In Sarsaparilla the neck emaciates and skin (in general) lies in folds.

Dr. E.B. Nash

SULPHUR: In other words, it seems to have the power of equalizing the circulation in persons subject to such local congestions and inflammations.

Dr. E.B. Nash

I treated in Gumpendorf Hospital at Viena, 57 cases of rheumatic carditis with one death and Spigelia was the only medicine employed.

Dr. Flaishman

A history of bed wetting in early life is a good pointer to Sepia.

Dr. T. Douglas Ross

The first great property of **Silicea** is its power over suppuration.

Dr. Hughes

Sulphur is to be considered in deep seated sepsis especially when associated with hectic fever and rigors.

Dr. D.M. Gibson

Every time she urinates she jumps from a sharp pain, as if a sharp instrument had been stuck under the great toenail, (Sulphur).

Dr. H.A. Roberts

Staphisagria is an excellent remedy for styes which is normally given when Pulsatilla fails. In my experience, I have found remedy affective in all cases of styes whether chronic or otherwise in lower or upper lids; recurrent styes.

Dr. R.B. Das

It is chiefly when scrofula manifests itself in the bones and joints that Silicea proves its remedy.

Dr. Hughes

The best remedy we have for small ulcers about the points of fingers is Sepia.

Dr. E.A. Farrington

We may use Sulphur in synovitis, particularly after exudation has taken place. Sulphur here produces absorption and very rapidly too, particularly in the knee.

Dr. E.A. Farrington

Senna is one of the best remedies in the Materia Medica for simple exhaustion with excessive nitrogenous waste.

Dr. E.A. Farrington

Silicea appears to cause a leucocytosis and may increase body resistance to disease in this way.

Dr. Ruddock

As for Silicea, this is cold blooded in chronic cases, but if a case of Silicea is acute or sub-acute, then it is ussally not blooded, warm blooded.

Dr. Ballokossy

I consider Stramonium the nearest similimum we have for hydrophobia.

Dr. George Royal

Bursitis: Sticta Pulminaria   has been found to be of great efficacy.

Dr. E.C. Price

Sepia   may be regarded as an excellent remedy for the paroxysms of hemicrania, which constitutes a source of distress to chlorotic females with lively temperaments.

Dr. Bochr

Sanguinaria   is decidedly homoeopathic in acute gastritis.

Dr. Deway

Saccharum Lactis   is a remdedy introduced by Dr. Swen. It was his 'Fatigue Powder,' the accuracy of which I have verfied.

Dr. Ying Ling

It is essential to ascertain the seat of the local disease with accuracy; for, every experianced homoeopath knows how in toothache for instance, it is necessary to select the remedy which in its provings has repeatedly acted upon the very tooth that suffers. The specific curative power of Sepia in those stubborn and sometimes fatal joint abscesses of the fingers and toes, in extraordinary conclusive evidence upon this point, for they differ from similar gatherings in location only, while the remedies so suitable for abscess elsewhere remain ineffectual here.

Dr. Boger

In Rachitis, caries and necrosis, Theridion, Curassavicum apprently goes to the root of the evil and destroys the cause.

Dr. Baruch

In many Psoric cases, the bowel nosodes are of great use and I think they are frequently neglected; most cases of migraine used one of the bowel nosodes to be cured permanently although Tuberculinum plays a great part here.

Dr. Quinton

Give Theridion gurassavicum for the vertigo and nausea associated with abscess of the liver.

Dr. Lippe

There are many people whose noses will begin to drip the minute they begin to eat, a fluent discharge from the nose. It is exceedingly annoying to the patient. I have a several occasions, been able to relieve that entirely by Trombidium.

Dr. H.A. Roberts

A person running down, never finding the right remedy, or relief only momentarily, has a constant desire to change, to travel, to go somewhere and do something different. That cosmopolitan condition of mind belongs strongly to the one who needs **Tuberculinum.**

Dr. Burnett.

I think in desperate cases of Jaundice in the newborn babies, Thyroidin will bring back the patient almost from the jaws of death.

Dr. Ghosh

I have cured probably 100 cases of Adenoids with Tuberculinum alcne.

Dr. J.T. Kent

I have wasted much time trying to find a remedy in cases with tuberculosis in the family. Now I like very much to augment Tuberculinum with Syphilinum.

Dr. Wilbur K. Bond

THUJA OCCIDENTALIS: Hahnemann recognized three miasms (as he called them) which complicated the treatment of all diseases. They were syphilis, psora and sycosis.

Sulphur was his chief anti-psoric, Mercury his anti-syphilitic and Thuja his anti-sycotic.

Whatever may be said against his theories along this line, certain it is that these three remedies do correct certain states of the system which seem to obstruct the curative action of other seemingly well-indicated remedies.

Dr. E.B. Nash

No home in town or country should be without stinging nettle tincture Urtica urens—if only because of its magic power over burns; for almost instant relief of pain and rapid healing. This applied of course to fairly superficial burns.

Dr. M.L. Tyler

Urtica Urems has cured obstinate cases of deltoid rheumatism in 10 drop doses of the tincture. It is thought this has the power to dissolve deposits of urates in the muscles.

Dr. Dewey

Vipera is the valuable remedy in brachia neuritis where it was noted that the patient supported the arm of the affected side to get relief.

Dr. Robert L. Redfield

Purnett termed **Vanadium** his 'sheet anchor' in fatty changes of the liver; also declares it meets the antheroma of the brain or liver to a nicety; real remedy of this organic change, and mentions Bellis Perennis as a complementary remedy. From slight experience with the remedy, this I can well believe. He claims that these two remedies have restored veritable physical wrecks to health.

Dr. Donnar

I would like to remind you of the efficacy of **Vinca Minor** in Alopecia areata. Hair fall out and are replaced by grey hair. Bald spots covered with a fine white wooly fuzz.

Dr. E.A. Farrington

Wiesbaden: By use of this remedy, the hair will grow rapidly and become darker in cases of falling of hair. Give in 200 dilution.

Dr. R.B. Das

16. SOME WIDER UNIVERSAL PRINCIPLES AND THE (CAUSE OF) UNCERTAIN RESULTS IN HOMOEOPATHY

(Also Relative Importance of Symptoms, Modalities and Clinical Experiences)

Ammonium Carb. has cured the cough of Influenza when everything else has failed, and I have more than once not found it necessary to give a second dose.

Dr. Younam

Tarentula or **Anthracinum** clear up the boils in a few days brilliantly and miraculously. (Hepar, Bell., Arn., Silicea.)

Dr. Dorothy Shephered

Actea Rac.: A woman will come to you with one a group of symptoms today and may come back to you with an entirely different group in a couple of weeks.

Dr. J.T. Kent

Hahnemann directs up to pay most attention to the symptoms of the mind, because the symptoms of the mind constitute the man himself. The highest and innermost symptoms are the most important, and these are the mind symptoms.

Dr. J.T. Kent

The mental symptoms can be classified in a remedy. The things that relate to the memory are not so imprtant as the things that relate to the intelligence are not so important as the things that relate to the affections or desire and avertions.

Dr. J.T. Kent

When the symptoms have been well gathered, the case is a
good as cured; it is easy then to find a remedy.

Dr. J.T. Ken

The capabilities of our Materia Medica are somethin
wonderful, but they could be developed much more rapidl
if a number of homoeopathic physicians would mak
application of the Materia Medica with accuracy an
intellegence, observing what they see and relating it literally

At the present day there is only a very small number c
homoeopathic physicians that can come together in a bod
and say things that are worth listening to, a shamefully sma
number when we consider the length of time Hahnemann'
books have been before the world.

Dr. J.T. Ken

Teething is a crisis and the things that are within will com
out all the time, just as there are troubles that are likely t
come out at the time of puberty and at the climacteric perioc

Dr. J.T. Ken

It is quite a profitable business for one who has not muc
conscience and not much intelligence. But a conscientiou
physician feels worried and knows he is not doing what h
ought to do to his patient, unless he reaches out for th
remedy which touches the constitution.

Dr. J.T. Ken

Homoeopathy is too often blamed when the blame lies in th
stupidity of the prescriber.

Dr. E.B. Nas

claim that he who prescribes, being guided by all the symptoms, will not and cannot fail, where a cure is at all possible. These are and must be our infalliable guides, or Similia, Similibus, Curantur is not true.

Dr. E.B. Nash

. remedy fits a general condition when the symptoms of that general condition are found in the remdy. Remember that, does so because all the symptoms agree.

Dr. J.T. Kent

Many a time have I seen hay fever wiped out in one season by a short-acting remedy, ony to return the next just the same, nd perhaps another remedy will be required. As soon as the hay fever is stopped you must begin with constitutional eatment. There will be symptoms, if you know how to hunt or them, that differ altogether from the acute attack.

Dr. J.T. Kent

While the patient himself with these deep related psoric ffections feels better gererally after the remedy, it will be months before his symptoms go away. He may say: "I feel etter, but my symptoms all appear to be here. I can eat better nd sleep better." Then it would be unwise to change the emedy.

Dr. J.T. Kent

ny remedy, of course, which corresponds to the totality of the symptoms is the remedy to administer.

Dr. J.T. Kent

All who do not perceive the difference between symptoms predicated of the patient and symptoms predicated of the parts will see that as only one symptom with the rest of them. When he takes up a case and works it out in the Repertory he will use it as one symptom. Yet that feature will sometimes rule out all the rest, because it is predicated of the patient and not predicated alone of his parts.

Dr. J.T. Kent

The medicines that are similar in general have to be compared, as to heat and cold. In that way we get a list of those that are ameliorated cold, and a list of those that are ameliorated by heat; and another non-descript list not ameliorated by either. That is the starting point, and we have to divide and subdivide these, and so on.

Dr. J.T. Kent

We sometimes do not discover this alternation of states until we have brought it back two or three times by incorrect prescribing.

Dr. J.T. Kent

I have never done better work with any other remedy in valvular diseases of the heart than Spongia.

Dr. E.B. Nash

Think what a state it is for a man who has been in good condition of health, respected in his business circles, to have a desire to commit suicide. The man's intellectual nature keeps the man in contact with the words; but his affections are largely kept to himself. A man can have affection for all sorts of things and perversion of the affections, but his intellect will guide him not to show his likes and dislikes to the world. The affections can not be seen, but man's intellect is subject to inspection. He cannot conceal his intellect.

Dr. J.T. Kent

AURUM MET: We shall see that the affections are interior, they are covered with a cloak, they are his innermost and are hidden from inspection; but the understanding is the outermost garment, it surrounds and hides his affections, just as does the garment he wears over the body hide the body. The affections that Aurm resembles are those like into the very innermost nature of man.

Dr. J.T. Kent

There must be no guess work in the study of provings. Every remedy must be used for its own symptoms, and for these there is no substitute. If a remedy does not work, the homoeopath can only examine the case a new and seek new symptoms and another remedy.

Dr. J.T. Kent

The medicine that covers the symptoms is the one that will change the economy from an abnormal to a normal state, and digestion will become orderly, and we will have growth and prosperity in the economy.

Dr. J.T. Kent

ACONITUM NEPELLUS: From fright vertigo comes on, or fainting; trembling; threatened abortion, or suppressed menstruation. Jaundice may be induced by it, and become chronic. There are other remedies for fright, prominent among which are Opium, Ignatia, Veratrum album, etc. Now in regard to the dry, cold air, no remedy has more prominently acute inflammations arising from dry, cold air. Nineteen out of twenty cases of croup arising from exposure to dry, cold air will be cured by Aconite.

Dr. E.B. Nash

AURUM METALLICUM: The Aurum patient is plunged into the deepest gloom and despair. Life is a burden, he desires death. Suicide dwells constantly in his mind. In men, I have observed it oftenest in connection with liver troubles. In women, with womb troubles, especially when enlarged, indurated or prolapsed. In both these cases, the result, so far as local conditions are concerned, seems to be from repeated attacks of congestion to the parts, which ends in hypertrophy.

Dr. E.B. Nash

ARSENICUM ALBUM: It makes little difference what the disease, if this persistant restlessness and especially if great weakness is also present, don't forget Arsenic.

Dr. E.B. Nash

ACONITUM NAPELLUS: So called homoeopaths have fallen into similar error by concluding that because Aconite did quickly cure in some cases having a high grade of fever, that therefore it was always the remedy with which to treat cases having high fever. They even fell into the routine habit of prescribing this remedy for the first stage of all inflammatory affections, and follow it with other remedies more appropriate to the whole case further on.

Dr. E.B. Nash

ARGENTUM NITRICUM: Unless the indications pointed

strongly to one in preference to the other remedy it might be well to try the vegetable first. The minerals are generally longer and deeper in their action, and would perhaps be preferable the more chronic the case.

Dr. E.B. Nash

AVENA SATIVA is prescribed in 10 to 20 drop doses of the tincture in a little water for its alleged tonic effect; numbness of the limbs as if paralysed is said to be symptom. It does seem to quiet the nervous system and bring about sleep; it like-wise relieves nervous headaches and fatigue most assuredly; it is to be preferred to the powerful coaltar drugs so constantly abused.

Dr. E.B. Nash

When Kali carb. fails, Anatherum may be tried in falling of hair from eyebrows.

Dr. R.B. Dash

You do not get all these things in the text, you have to see them applied but the things that I give you that are brought out clinically are those things that have come from applying the symptoms of the remedy at the bed side of the sick folks.

Dr. J.T. Kent

In sleeplessness from anxiety, restlessness, anguish, fear, when man, woman or child tosses feverishly in despair of ever getting off to sleep, Aconite is simply scientific magic.

Dr. M.L. Tyler

When the symptoms seem to point out a particular remedy

12

with which the modalities however do not agree; it is only negatively indicated, and the physician has the most urgent reasons to doubt its fitness; he should therefore seek for another having the same symptoms.

Dr. Boger

When there are papillae on the tip of the tongue the child has worms, Cina is the remedy.

Dr. Edwards

No remedy should be given on one symptom. Study the remedy and disease thoroughly to ascertain if the two are similar to each other to expect to a cure. Any deviation from that rule is ruinous and will lead to the practice of giving medicines on single symptom.

Dr. J.T. Kent

Do not dwell upon the cancer for it is not the cancer but the patient that you are treating. It is the patient that is sick, and whenever a patient is sick enough to have a cancer, his state of order is too much disturbed to be cured.

Dr. J.T. Kent

The physician's knowledge as to what he is doing is his own, and the greatest comfort he can get out of it, is his own. He never expect that anyone will appreciate what he has done or what he has avoided. The physician who desires praise and sympathy for what he has done generally has no conscience.

Dr. J.T. Ken

If it be necessary in the case of a very sensitive patient, t employ the smallest possible dose and to bring about the most rapid result, one single olfaction merely of a single globule the size of a mustard seed will suffice.

Dr. Hahnemann

In old workmen, labourers, and the over worked and flagged, Bellis perennis is a princely remedy.

Dr. Burnett

Symphytum follows Arnica will if pricking pain and soreness of periosteum remains after an injury.

Dr. H.C. Allen

Many of the ovarian or tubular symptoms that develop during menses are dependent on sycosis.

Dr. H.A. Roberts

The psoric patient has many uncomfortable sensations, such as sharp cutting, neuralgic pains about the heart; those patients think they are about to die and want to lie down and keep quiet but there is no danger; it is the sycotic and syphilitic heart patients who die and then suddenly without warning.

Dr. H.A. Roberts

Any case of cancer complicated by a weak heart or diseased kidneys can hardly get well, because the reaction to curative remedy will kill such a patient in a comparatively short time.

Dr. A.H. Grimmer

No drug will do equally well for another curatively, while

several may be more or less palliative, which is quite another matter.

Dr. M.L. Tyler

Never think that homoeopathy can cure everything; it cannot. But it can relieve even the incurable to such an extent that it is difficult to realise, at times its incurability.

Dr. M.L. Tyler

It is a prime rule not to keep repeating your remedy when the intervals between aggravations of the disease are lengthening. This is an indication that the patient is improving.

Homoeo. Recorder, Aug. 31

The so-called germ diseases: They cannot thrive in the blood or tissues if the organism is not primarily sick and affords a suitable soil for them. In health, immunity from germs is well known. When such an immunity is absent, health is likewise absent; under the circumstances, it becomes the duty of the true physician to remove that susceptibility of the organism to germs and other disease influences which constitutes the primary factor in so-called zymotic diseases.

Dr. Younan

In acute troubles, if it is possible to wait the time through for the remedy, give it very high at the close of the attack and you will be very likely to so build up that constitution that the next attack will be much lighter.

Dr. J.T. Ken

High fever, great pain, great fear, strong fits of anger, o

emotional excitement shorten the action of a remedy and indicate repetition.

Dr. Pierre Schmidt

When notwithstanding the carefully chosen remedy and the patient's faultless diet, the sick condition on the contrary, is not at all changed, the cause usually lies in want of receptivity which we must sick to remove either by repeated small doses or by medicines recommended for deficient reaction.

Dr. Boger

It has been frequently, the writers experience that patients who are slow to react to remedies have children with similar peculiarities and in such cases, repeated doses are much likely to be needed.

Dr. Hardy

If keynotes are taken as final and the general do not conform, then will come to failures.

Dr. M.L. Tyler

Failure to diagnose may wreck the physician while diagnosis without the remedy is poor consolation for the patient.

Dr. M.L. Tyler

If inward affections work outward towards the surface there is not usually cause for alarm, but if they go the other way look out for breakers, there is shipwreck ahead.

Dr. E.B. Nash

BARYTA CARB: One thing in homoeopathy taught in

Hahnemann's Organon is that unless there are symptoms to indicate the remedy, no great things should be expected from the administration of the remedy.

Dr. J.T. Kent

BRYONIA ALBA: The urine is scanty and only exceptionally (or as I would express it reactionally) copious. We must remember that every remedy has a dual action. These two actions are termed primary and secondary. I think that the so-called secondary action is only the reaction of the organism against the first or primary (so-called) action of the drug. For instance, the real action of Opium is to produce sleep or stupor, the reaction is wakefulness; of Podophyllum, Aloes, etc., catharsis; the reaction constipation, and I think that the truly homoeopathic curative must be in accord with the primary (so-called) effects of every drug in order to get the best and most radical cure, but if given for the secondary (so-called) symptoms, the primary ones having passed by, we should carefully inquire for all the symptoms which have preceded those which are present; and taking both past and present, let them all enter into the picture whose counterpart is to be found in the drug which is to cure. Any other method is only palliative and not curative.

Dr. E.B. Nash

CALADIUM: You can only cure these patients if they desire to reform, and if you can inspire them to live a better life. Without this you cannot save them, and those who take delight in such things are not worth saving, and medicine will not take hold of them. To cure, the patient must use his will to help the remedy.

Dr. J.T. Kent

CALCAREA SULPH: Most inveterate catarrh of the nose has been cured by this remedy.

Dr. J.T. Kent

CALCAREA CARB: It is a strange thing to see a bright little girl 8 or 9 years old taking on sadness, melancholy, and commencing to talk about the future world, and the angels, and that she wants to die and go there, and she is sad, and wants to read the Bible all day. That is a strange thing; and yet Calcarea has cured that.

Dr. J.T. Kent

CALCAREA CARB: Suppose the patient always avoided warm things and much clothing, and wanted the cold open air, and still had a dozen key-notes, you would find every time that Calcarea would fail.

Dr. J.T. Kent

CALCAREA SULPH: This is a valuable remedy for catarrh of bladder, with copious yellow pus. It has cured chronic inflammation of the kidney.

Dr. J.T. Kent

CAPSICUM: Most of the substances that are used on the table as seasoning in foods will in the course of a generation or two be very useful medicines, because people poison themselves with these substances, tea, coffee, pepper, and these poisonous affects in the parents cause in the children a predisposition to disease, which is similar to the disease produced by these substances.

Dr. J.T. Kent

CUPRUM MET: A drink of water seems to flow through the bowel with a gurgle.

Dr. J.T. Kent

CAPSICUM: An impulse is sometimes overwhelming and over balances the mind, and he commits suicide. Some persons lie awake at night and long for death, and there is no reason for it. That is the state of the will, insanity of the will. Desires are of the will; impulses come into the thoughts. If he desires to have a knife to commit suicide, that is altogether different from an impulse to commit suicide.

Dr. J.T. Kent

CAPSICUM: If the patient has a good constitutional state he will get over the cold on the acute remedy, but the old gouty, rheumatic, flabby patients need a constitutional remedy.

Dr. J.T. Kent

CARBO VEGETABILIS: The woman feels best when she has more or less of a leucorrhoeas-it seems a sort of protection. These discharges that we meet every day are dried up and controlled by local treatments, by washes, and by local applications of every kind-and the patient put into the hands of the undertaker, or made a miserable wreck. If these catarrhal patients are not healed from within out, the discharges had better be allowed to go on. While these discharges exit the patient is comfortable.

Dr. J.T. Kent

COLOCYNTHIS: You will seldom find this medicine indicated in strong, vigorous, healthy people who have suddenly become sick. *Dr. J.T. Kent*

CARBO VEGETABILIS: The study of the faces of remedies is very profitable. It is profitable to study the faces of healthy people that you may be able to judge their intentions from their facial expressions. A man shows his business of life in his face; he shows his method of thinking, his hatreds, his longings, and his loves. How easy it is to pick out a man who has never loved to do anything but to eat-the Epicurean face. How easy it is to pick out a man who has never loved anything but money-the miserly face. You can see the love in many of the professional faces; you can single out the student's face. These are only manifestations of the love of the life which they live. some manifest hatred; hatred of the life in which they have been forced to live; hatred of mankind; hatred of life. In those who have been disappointed to everything they have undertaken to do we see hatred stamped upon the face. We see these things in remedies just as we see them in people.

Dr. J.T. Kent

CARBO VEGETABILIS: The children that grow up under the care of the homoeopathic physician will never have consumption, or Bright's disease; they are all turned into order and they will die of old age, or be worn out properly by business cares; they will not rush out. It is the duty of the physician to watch the little ones. To save them from their inheritances and their downward tendencies is the greatest work of his life. That is worth living for. When we see these tendencies cropping out in the little ones we should never intimate that they are due to the father or mother.

Dr. J.T. Kent

CAUSTICUM: Dryness of the mouth and throat; rawness of the throat, must swallow constantly on account of a sensation of fulness in the throat, a nervous feeling in the throat. This is often a fore-runner of paralysis.

Dr. J.T. Kent

CARBO VEGETABILIS: The physician's knowledge as to what he is doing in his own, and the greatest comfort he can get out of it is his own. He needs never expect that anyone will appreciate what he has done, or what he has avoided. The physician who desires praise and sympathy for what he has done generally has no conscience. The noble, upright, truthful physician works in the night; he works in the dark; he works quietly; he is not seeking for praise.

Dr. J.T. Kent

COCCULUS INDICUS: It is entirely without inflammation. It is a sort of a paralytic stiffness, a paralysis of the tired body and mind. The Cocculus headaches and backaches, pains and distress are present. A man will stretch out his leg on a chair and he cannot flex it until he reaches down with his hands to assist.

Dr. J.T. Kent

CUPRUM METALLICUM: During the progress of the labour the patient suddenly becomes blind. All light seems to her to disappear from the room, the labor pains cease, and convulsions come on, commencing in the fingers and toes. When you meet these cases do not forget Cuprum.

Dr. J.T. Kent

FERRUM MET: Woman suffers much from haemorrhage from the uterus, especially during and after the climacteric period.

Dr. J.T. Kent

CUPRUM MET: The individual has become debilitated and worn out with excitement, but this discharge barely kept him dive. He has gradually grown weaker, but he has kept about because he had a discharge. It has furnished him and safety-valve. If stopped suddenly covulsions will come on.

Dr. J.T. Kent

CALCAREA CARB: It has no such tearing down nature in it. It does not establish inflammation around foreign bodies and tends to support them out, but causes a fibrous deposit around bullets and other foreign substances in the flesh. It causes tubercular deposits to harden and contract and become encysted.

Dr. J.T. Kent

DIGITALIS: When a patient goes to sleep the cerebrum says to the cerebellum: "Now you carry on this breathing a little while, I am getting tired." But the cerebellum is not equal to the occasion. It is congested, and just as soon as the cerebrum begins to rest the cerebellum goes to sleep, too, and lets the patient suffer; and in that way we get suffocation. The cerebellum presides over respiration during sleep and the cerebrum presides over respiration when the patient is awake. We might learn that from the provings of medicines if we never found it before.

Dr. J.T. Kent

IGNATIA: Thirst when you would not expect it. Thirst during chill, but none during the fever, if she has a feverish state.

Dr. J.T. Kent

DULCAMARA: Every experienced physician must have met with many cases where for a time he felt unable to cope with the case because of his inability to reach the constitutional state that underlies this continual taking cold. So he puzzles, for a long time, and prescribes on the immediate attack and palliates it.

Dr. J.T. Kent

FERRUM MET: She is feeble, she suffers from palpitation and dyspnoea, she has great weakness with inability to do anything like work, she feels that she must lie down yet the face is flushed. This is called a pseudo-plethora.

Dr. J.T. Kent

FERRUM MET: Green sickness: "Ferrum will be found of great value-when the symptoms agree-in that wonderful anaemic state called "green sickness," that comes on with girls at the time of puberty and in the years that follow it. There will be almost no menstrual flow, but a cough will develop, with great pallor. So common is this sickness among girls that all mothers are acquainted with and dread it.

Dr. J.T. Kent

GELSEMIUM: may not have produced erysipelas, it will stop the progress of the disease in a few hours, and the patient will go to a quick recovery. If we master thoroughly the Materia Medica, we do not stop to see if a remedy produces certain kinds of inflammation, etc., but we consider the state of the patient.

Dr. J.T. Kent

HYOSCYAMUS: When the patient is ill natured, unreasonable and complains beyond all reason, in rheumatism, or any other disease, a few dose of Hyoscyamus 3x will surprise you very pleasantly.

Dr. Cuthburt

HEPAR SULPH: The leucorrhoea is so copious that she is compelled to wear a napkins, and the napkin, I have been told by women who have been cured by Hepar, are so offensive that they must be taken away and washed at once because the odour permeates the room.

Dr. J.T. Kent

IGNATIA: A sensitive girl, though she would not let anyone but her mother knows of it, falls in love with a married man. She lies awake nights, sobs. She says, "Mother, why do I cannot keep that man out of my mind."

Dr. J.T. Kent

IGNATIA: We do not know half as much about the human mind as we think we do. We only know its manifestations. These little things belong to this sphere of action of this medicine. The one who knows the Materia Medica applies it in its breadth and its length, and sees in it that which is similar.

Dr. J.T. Kent

IODINE Iodine has the impulse to kill, not from anger, not from my sense of justice, but without any cause.

Dr. J.T. Kent

A Natrum sulph. patient will say, "Doctor, you do not know how I have to resist killing myself. An impulse to do it comes into my mind.

Dr. J.T. Kent

KALI CARB: The capabilities of our Materia Medica are something wonderful, but they could develop much more rapidly if a number of homoeopathic physicians would make application of the Materia Medica with accuracy and intelligence, observing what they see and relating it literally. At the present day there is only a very small number of homoeopathic physicians that can come together in a body and say things that are worth listening to, a shamefully small number when we consider the length of time Hahnemann's books have been before the world.

Dr. J.T. Kent

MEDORHINUM: The husband's history give the cause, and this remedy will cure.

Dr. J.T. Kent

Remember **Causticum** in those difficult rheumatoid cases of Arthritis where there are deformities and contractions, and the patient suffers more in cold, dry winds and less in warm wet days.

Dr. M.L. Tyler